A theoretical framework for clinical specialist nursing:

An example from diabetes

To Mom and Dad and to Eva, Peter and Richard—no words could ever describe how much you mean to me

A theoretical framework for clinical specialist nursing:
An example from diabetes

S Llahana

APS Publishing, Fivepin Limited, 91 Crane Street, Salisbury, Wiltshire, UK, SP1 2PU

British Library Cataloguing in Publication Data
A catalogue record for this book is available from the British Library.

ISBN 1 9038773 6 9

Printed in the United Kingdom by Lightning Source, Milton Keynes

Contents

Acknowledgements

The greatest thanks and sincere appreciation go to my mentors, Professor Vivien Coates and Professor Brenda Poulton, for their continuous support and intellectual guidance without which this work might otherwise had been an impossible task. Special thanks go to Anne Hagan for her assistance in reviewing this book. I would like to thank Professor Ann Hamric for her valuable suggestions in this study, especially regarding the CNS role development section—her work inspired me and provided the basis for this book. I am very grateful to all the diabetes specialist nurses working in the UK and the nurses, physicians and people with diabetes from Greece who participated in this study. The study exploring the CNS role presented in this book was funded by the Greek State Scholarship Foundation and was undertaken at the University of Ulster in Northern Ireland.

I would also like to express my appreciation to my manager, Maia-Lisa Rand, for her support and for allowing me the time to write this book. Finally, but not least, I would like to thank Dr Gerard Conway for his assistance in developing my CNS role; I feel highly privileged to be working with such a supportive and inspirational consultant.

Preface

The role of the clinical nurse specialist (CNS) has been defined as advanced, flexible and multifaceted. The CNS role was established in North America in the early 1960s but its implementation in the United Kingdom only started in the late 1970s. The CNS role is the most debated of all the advanced practice nursing roles, and has generated considerable discussion and controversy. This is because the many sub-roles, activities and skills of the CNS make their role expanded, versatile, and unique, but at the same time contribute to the confusion surrounding the CNS practice. In addition, the role performance of a CNS is influenced by a number of organisational and personal factors, as well as expectations from different parties with whom the CNSs collaborate in their practice.

There is a wide range of theoretical and empirical literature in relation to the CNS role especially from America, mostly published in journal articles. However, the studies undertaken to explore the CNS role have only examined partial aspects of this role and there has been no empirical research to encompass an in-depth exploration of this role. Similarly, limited evidence exists on factors that enhance or inhibit the CNS role development and implementation.

The aim of this book is to bridge this gap in the nursing literature by undertaking a comprehensive in-depth exploration of all aspects of the CNS role, underpinned by a firm theoretical framework. A thorough review of the existing literature regarding the CNS role and a nationwide study in the United Kingdom were undertaken for this purpose. The study involved 334 CNSs working in the area of diabetes. The concepts relevant to the CNS role were identified, explored and construed in a validated theoretical framework derived from the Role Theory field. Although the sample of the study involved diabetes specialist nurses (DSNs), the findings can be generalised to the wider population of CNSs. The CNS role theoretical framework explored in this book can underpin the study of any CNS role, independent of their speciality, and explains the CNS role development and performance.

The book is primarily intended for clinical nurse specialists but can be of great interest to other advanced nurse practitioners and general nurses, as well as nurse administrators, educators and nursing students. A detailed exploration of the development of the instrument used to study the CNS role is undertaken by including a description of the study methods, data analysis and results. This aims to provide the researcher undertaking similar studies with a useful guide in selecting and applying methods appropriate to their research questions. All chapters of this book are underpinned by the same theoretical framework and are interconnected. However, each can stand on its own by exploring a specific and unique aspect of the CNS role.

Diabetes nursing as a speciality is a particular clinical nursing speciality and the DSN and CNS roles follow the same principles. Therefore, the term 'CNS' in this book includes that of the DSN. The use of the term 'DSN' denotes that the literature cited considers exclusively the role of the DSN. This term is also used to refer to respondents in the present study and its findings.

The comprehensive exploration of each individual CNS concept and the validation of the CNS role theoretical framework are undertaken in the first seven chapters. The difference between specialisation in an area of nursing and nursing speciality, the role characteristics of the CNS and evolution of the CNS role in North America and the United Kingdom are explored in Chapter 1. The development and definition of the DSN role in the UK are presented in the second part of this chapter. Chapter 2 discusses the relevance of role theory to nursing and the development of the theoretical framework underpinning the exploration of the CNS role. The CNS role-related concepts, Personal Characteristics and Skills, Work and Organisational Factors, Role Development and Role Performance, were explored in a UK study involving DSNs and are discussed in Chapters 3 to 6 respectively.

Chapter 7 examines the associations between the above role concepts. A validated theoretical framework was developed, which, although focused on the DSN role, can guide the exploration of the CNS role and explains the interrelations between the factors that influence role performance and development. This chapter also discusses the strengths and limitations of the present study exploring the CNS role and its implications for nursing practice. The final chapter provides a perspective from a European country—Greece—where the CNS role has not yet been introduced. It explores the feasibility of implementing this role in the clinical setting and identifies barriers and obstacles to its implementation, as well as strategies to overcome these.

Foreword

This book is timely as the number of clinical specialist nurses, in the UK, is rapidly increasing. Furthermore, the Nursing and Midwifery Council (NMC) in its role in public protection is, at the time of writing, reviewing specialist nursing and higher-level practice beyond initial registration. The Council clearly sets out the characteristics of nurses with an advanced level of knowledge and competence and this book will go further in informing that debate. By using Hamric and Taylor's framework for the development of clinical nurse specialists, Sofia demonstrates that the role of the specialist nurse is not static. The findings of the research reported in this book can be applied to educational programmes preparing specialist nurses and also for supporting specialist nurses in post. It should be an essential text for those wishing to understand the complexities of specialist nurses and all the attendant titles.

Professor Brenda Poulton

Professor Vivien Coates

University of Ulster
April 2005

1

Evolution and definition of the clinical nurse specialist in the USA and in the UK

1.1 Introduction

Specialisation in nursing infers a narrowing of the range of work to be done and an increase in depth of knowledge and skills. The setting up of the first training school in nursing by Florence Nightingale, after the Crimean War, can be considered as the starting point for specialisation. The publication of her work 'Notes on nursing: what it is and what it is not', which was directed mainly towards professional nurses, also contributed to the establishment of specialist and advanced nursing practice (Castledine, 1998a).

This chapter presents a brief description of the evolution of the clinical nurse specialist (CNS) role in the USA and the UK. In addition, the distinction between clinical specialist nursing and specialisation in nursing is discussed, and the role and characteristics of the CNS defined. The final part of this chapter discusses the evolution and definition of the role of the diabetes specialist nurse (DSN) in the United Kingdom.

1.2 Evolution of the role of the clinical nurse specialist

1.2.1 Evolution of the role of the clinical nurse specialist in North America

Nightingale was the first to distinguish between two separate classes of nurses, the amateur, hired, domestic servant and the professionally prepared hospital nurse. Although Nightingale did not mention the term 'clinical specialist' in her writings, she introduced some concepts basic to the role. She was respected for her clinical, administrative and teaching skills. She was assertive and knew how to find and use power. Moreover, she urged nurses to ally themselves with physicians in order to reach the objective of caring for wounded soldiers (Nightingale, 1859).

The concept of the nurse specialist was first documented in the *American Journal of Nursing* by an American private duty nurse, describing specialists in three areas: surgical, paediatric and obstetrical nursing (De Witt, 1900). Designation was given to nurses who had graduated from specialised hospitals or private-duty nurses who limited their practice to the care of particular types of patients. De Witt's perception of specialisation was congruent with the long experience of a nurse in nursing practice. She noted that nurses became so adept in a particular area they considered themselves 'specialists'.

In the first half of the twentieth century, the terms 'specialism' and 'specialist nursing' were restricted to knowledge and skills associated with a particular medical condition or disease. Up until the late 1960s, nurse education was geared towards preparing and sustaining nurse generalists in limited functional specialities. Moreover, due to the lack of formal educational courses on specialisation, it would be difficult to say that these nurses developed specialist nursing skills; rather they were just good generalists who adapted well to medical task work (Castledine, 1994). White (1977; p41) criticised this when she wrote:

> *'As a profession we expect ourselves to know everything and if we continue to feel that the general trained nurse must know it all, we shall continue to be a profession which is broadly based in knowledge, but sadly lacking in depth.'*

To overcome these limitations of nurses' educational preparation, Johnson (1962; p99) suggested the development of programmes where professional nurses would:

> *'...need to think, to solve problems, to make decisions, and to use knowledge and imagination in developing creative and original approaches in nursing care. ...Educational emphasis also is placed on the patient as a person requiring individualised care.'*

As a solution, Johnson suggested the introduction of clinical nurse specialists into nursing service. Reiter (1966) used the term 'nurse clinician' to refer to the nurse whose role would be to demonstrate and provide nursing care, plan and supervise patient care given by other nurses, and serve as staff consultant and educator. She asserted that organised graduate education programmes represent the most efficient means of preparing such practitioners.

While specialisation initially referred to the long experience of the nurse in a specific speciality, the role of the CNS, as Hamric (1998; p57) emphasised, '...was clearly developed to improve the quality of nursing care delivery by bring a nurse with specialized experience and advanced formal education to the direct care interface'.

As early as 1952, the National League for Nursing (USA) proposed that the Baccalaureate programme should prepare the nurse for general professional nursing and the Master's programme for specialisation (Castledine, 1994). In the late 1960s in the United States, it had become generally recognised that a clinical nursing speciality was not only a designation for an expert clinician, but that graduate preparation in a specified area of clinical nursing was also an essential requisite. Furthermore, developing nursing clinical education at the graduate level would increase the professional status of nursing (Sparacino, 1986). In the early 1980s, the American Nurses Association (ANA) issued a Policy Statement (ANA, 1980) (cited in Keeling and Bigbee, 2005), which clearly delineated the criteria required to enter the CNS role. These included educational preparation at graduate level (Master's or Doctorate) and specialty certification through nursing's professional society. ANA also announced that specialisation in nursing was clearly established and indicative of the advancement of the nursing profession. By 1984 in the United States, there were 129 accredited programmes preparing clinical nurse specialists at Master's level (Hamric, 1989).

In 1996, the American Association of Colleges of Nursing published T*he Essentials of Master's Education for Advanced Practice Nursing* which provided a nationally agreed blueprint for graduate nursing programmes, recommending a core curriculum common to all Master's students (Sparacino, 2005).

1.2.2 Evolution of the role of the clinical nurse specialist in the United Kingdom

The role of the CNS in the UK evolved much later than that in the USA and Canada, and has still not been clearly defined. Nevertheless, its evolution was very much influenced by the American model of clinical specialist nursing. The Nurses' Registration Act of 1919, which was the first type of specialisation in nursing in the UK, identified four specialities: sick children, mental nursing, care of the mentally handicapped, and fever nursing (Castledine, 1982). The development of degree programmes was a more recent event than in the USA, and Manchester University was the first to offer a Master's degree in clinical specialist nursing in the late 1970s (Castledine, 1998a).

Castledine (1982) undertook the first research study in the UK aiming to identify clinical nurse specialists in England and Wales, as defined by themselves and/or senior nursing management or health authorities. In addition, the study aimed to compare the development of their role with that of CNSs in the USA. The method of identifying participants was carried out by writing to the press, the Royal College of Nursing, and other specialist nurse interest groups. An appeal was made to nurses who held the title of CNS to contact the researcher.

The study identified 353 CNSs, of whom 49 were self-defined. Only 8% of the participants came significantly near to fulfilling the role of the CNS, but none held all the essential characteristics of the role. Regarding the educational preparation for undertaking the role, only two of the 353 nurses held a Master's degree in clinical nursing. Moreover, the amount and type of management and research activities these nurses were involved in were very limited. Castledine (1982) found that the development and progress of CNSs in England and Wales were influenced by those of CNSs in North America. However, he concluded that in the early 1980s the CNS role was still confined to the medical profession's model of areas for specialisation.

In recent years in the UK, although education at Master's level is not a prerequisite for a CNS, the nurse is required to undertake additional specialist preparation, and have experience and educational qualifications at first degree level. Programmes of specialist education concentrate on four broad areas: clinical practice, care and programme management, clinical practice development, and clinical practice leadership (Castledine, 1995a).

1.2.2.1 The influence of different professional organisations on the CNS role evolution

It is apparent that in the past three decades in the UK, the career pathway and structure for CNSs have been greatly debated. Individual groups within nursing, as Castledine (1998b; p38) maintained, '...have given a great deal of thought to issues such as how to describe clinical expertise and development and what title to give clinical developers.' The publication of different reports and documents contributed to the development of clinical specialist practice. More specifically, the document on career pathways, published by the Department of Health in 1995, highlighted the factors that influence career development and diversity of available career roles and opportunities for qualified practitioners, employers and educationalists (Castledine, 1998b).

The Government has also acknowledged the development and advancement in nursing roles. It is noted in the document *The New NHS: Modern, Dependable* that: '...expert nurses are taking on a leadership role, mentoring and educating nurses and other staff, managing care, developing nurse-led clinics and district wide services' (Department of Health, 1997; p46). This document gave CNSs many opportunities to advance and clarify their role.

The Royal College of Nursing (RCN) has promoted the importance of a clinical career structure for nurses for more than 20 years. In 1988, the RCN published a report which described the development of specialities in nursing, and defined the role of the CNS and its components (Royal College of Nursing, 1988).

The foundation of the United Kingdom Central Council for Nursing, Midwifery and Health Visiting (UKCC)—currently known as the Nursing and Midwifery Council (NMC)—in 1979 was, among others, an essential movement in the development and expansion of clinical specialist nursing (Castledine, 1994). The document *The Scope of Professional Practice* (UKCC, 1992a) maintained that professional practice requires the application of knowledge and the simultaneous exercise of judgement and skill, which takes place in a context of continuing change and development. It also recommended that accountability and the range of responsibilities for individual professionals be related to their personal experience, knowledge, education and skills.

Later, in the PREP (Post-Registration Education and Practice) document, it was asserted that professional practice alone following registration is not enough to meet additional specialist needs; further education is required for effective and safe practice. It was also noted in this document that CNSs are the practitioners who are able to exercise higher levels of judgement and discretion in clinical care (UKCC, 1994). However, unlike the USA where a Master's degree is a requisite for entering the CNS role, in the UK educational standards are less clearly defined and qualification for the role tends to depend largely on a nurse's level of clinical experience and management discretion. With the increasing emphasis on academic and clinical credibility, and as specialist practice requires '...higher levels of judgement, discretion and decision-making in clinical care' (UKCC, 1998; p1), educational preparation of the CNS at Master's level is becoming imperative.

Formal accreditation of specialist nursing is another burning issue in the UK; that is, there is no official recognition and approval for CNSs who undertake substantial professional learning and acquire additional clinical competence. In the USA, CNSs generally are expected to hold a recognised advanced practice certification within a specialty, although this expectation is problematic for CNSs in specialties without such examinations (Hamric, 2005). In the UK, however, the CNSs (including DSNs discussed in the next section), although required to be registered with the NMC in order to practics, do not have professional certification for their speciality. This is expected to change, given the implementation of the Agenda for Change in 2005 in the National Health Service (NHS). This initiative aims to evaluate and accredit nursing roles based on a nationally agreed *Knowledge and Skills Framework* (Department of Health, 2004), which may involve certification by examination. A Master's level of education for advanced practice nursing, which includes CNSs, is also recommended.

1.3 Definition of the role of the clinical nurse specialist

1.3.1 The difference between specialisation in nursing and nursing speciality

Before attempting to define the role of the CNS, it is essential to make a distinction between nurse specialists and nurses working in a speciality. The Royal College of Nursing (1988; p5) defines nursing speciality as:

> '...*a component of the whole field of nursing, usually identified by being concerned with an age, sex or population group (for example midwifery or paediatric nursing), a body system (such as renal nursing), a health or status situation (for instance health visiting), a method of investigation (for example endoscopy or screening) or another aspect of nursing. Specialities are derived from the major branches of nursing care: mental handicap; mental health; care of the adult; care of the child; and midwifery.*'

On the other hand, specialisation (specialism) in nursing may have its roots in one or more of the above branches, but the role of the specialist nurse is determined by function rather than by the setting in which it is performed. Specialisation in nursing, therefore, implies a deeper level of knowledge, skills and qualifications in a particular field of nursing care than the one that is acquired during general training. However, the Royal College of Nursing (1988; p6) asserts that 'this does not make the nurse specialist', and goes further to define CNSs as:

> '...*experts in a particular aspect of nursing care—they are nurses prepared beyond the level of registration. They demonstrate refined clinical practice, either as a result of significant experience or advanced expertise, or knowledge in a branch or speciality.*'

Hamric (2005) noted that advanced practice nursing includes not only specialisation, but it also involves expansion and advancement. The American Nurses Association (1984) defined specialisation as a narrow focus on a part of the whole field of nursing, which requires the application of a broad range of theories to selected nursing phenomena. This secures depth of understanding as a basis for advances in nursing. The reduction in the range of knowledge expected of nurse specialists results in the development of the depth of knowledge and skills that can be applied directly in the clinical setting to enhance patient care. Therefore, as Wade and Moyer (1989) characteristically stated, clinical nurse specialists know more and more about less and less.

1.3.2 Role characteristics and definition of the clinical nurse specialist

Originally, the CNS role developed to provide an expert practitioner service at the bedside of the patient. Today, the role of the CNS has expanded beyond the hospital setting, with a client-based focus (Beecroft and Papenhausen, 1989). Hamric (1989) states that regardless of setting, CNS practice should be directed toward improving patient care and nursing practice. Moreover, CNSs must be able to influence the quality of nursing care in a larger group of patients than they can personally attend. If the CNS does not maintain clinical practice and a focus on patients/clients and their families, that individual ceases to be a CNS and should not be allowed to use this title (Holt, 1984).

The role of the CNS from its inception was firmly grounded in clinical practice. However, since the earliest days, the role included other components such as education, consultation and research, besides direct patient care (Georgopoulos and Christman, 1970). The CNSs role is multifaceted and very complex, and therefore their practice is flexible and changes in response to the needs of patients and/or institutions. Almost 30 years before Hamric, Hellman (1974; p167) maintained that the CNS role is a flexible one and, therefore, must have a flexible definition. She noted that:

> *'The generalities of the role can be defined and communicated, and they express the commonalities among all such practitioners, regardless of specialty. But the specifics of the role can only be defined in the context of the individual practitioner in her particular setting and in her time.'*

Great confusion exists with the proliferation of nursing titles and roles following registration, especially in the UK. In the American literature the generic term 'advanced practice nursing' encapsulates all the various advanced clinical nursing roles, such as clinical nurse specialist, nurse practitioner, nurse consultant, nurse clinician, including that of the clinical nurse specialist, certified nurse-midwife, and nurse case manager (Hamric, 2005). In the UK, however, although there is agreement on the core skills and competences as well as qualifications of graduate nurses, advanced practice is viewed as independent of the clinical specialist practice (Castledine, 2003). The UKCC (1990) report on post-registration education endorsed two concepts of practice development following registration as a nurse: clinical specialist nurse and advanced nurse practitioner.

In this book, the author has adopted the definition by Hamric (2005; p89) and views clinical specialist nursing as part of the 'advanced practice nursing'; this is:

> *'...the application of an expanded range of practical, theoretical, and research-based competencies to phenomena experienced by patients within a specialized clinical area of the larger discipline of nursing.'*

Hamric (2005) identified three primary criteria which must be met before a nurse can be considered an advanced practice nurse (including the CNS). These include graduate education at Master's or Doctoral level, professional certification for practice at an advanced level within a nursing speciality, and practice focused on patients and their families, with direct clinical practice as a central focus.

When explored independently of other advanced practice nursing roles, the role of the CNS has been described as advanced, complex, multifaceted and flexible in response to the needs of patients and/or institutions. It includes the following components (sub-roles): expert practice, consultation, education, research, and management (Hamric and Spross, 1989; Humphris, 1994a; McGee, 1998; Sparacino and Cooper, 1990). Newer work has focused on core competencies of clinical specialist nursing, which include: direct clinical practice, expert coaching and guidance, consultation, research, clinical and professional leadership, collaboration, and ethical decision-making (Sparacino, 2005). In addition, the National Association of Clinical Nurse Specialists (NACNS) in the USA has further defined the CNS role as practice in three spheres of influence: the patient/client sphere, the nurse/nursing practice sphere, and the organisation/system sphere (NACNS, 2004).

1.4 The role of the diabetes specialist nurse in the United Kingdom

1.4.1 Evolution of the role of the diabetes specialist nurse

Diabetes nurses have been around for more than 70 years, following the discovery of insulin. A painting in the entrance hall of the Joslin Centre in Boston, USA, depicting a nurse seated beside a child, and demonstrating an insulin injection, shows clearly the early understanding of diabetes nursing (MacKinnon, 1998b). In the UK, Walker (1953; p447) was the first to point out the need for nurses to specialise in diabetes and noted that:

> *'The need for field work in the care and aftercare of the diabetic patient becomes apparent the longer one works in a central clinic. It is doubtful whether the family doctor can find time to undertake all this work. Teaching the diabetic has to be slow, painstaking, and above all consistent. ...This work can be done by a woman* [nurse] *of the right personality who must have considerable tact as well as expert knowledge.'*

As early as the 1950s, a diabetes specialist health visitor was appointed at the Leicester Royal Infirmary. The role was mainly concerned with patients' direct expert care and education in the diabetes clinic or at their homes. It also included teaching and information sessions on diabetes for school teachers and day-care staff in facilities attended by children with diabetes. This role was also extended to visits and provision of advice and consultation to people working with adults with diabetes in their employment setting. The diabetes specialist health visitor kept records of her visits and acted as a co-ordinator of patient information within the diabetes team and for other health professionals. Facilitating collaboration of care between primary and secondary care was also part of her role (Walker, 1953). It can be seen that the role of the diabetes specialist health visitor, as described by Walker, included a number of activities which, even after almost 50 years, form the basic functions of the DSN role.

Although the appointment of the diabetes specialist health visitor proved beneficial in the care of patients with diabetes (Walker, 1953), it was not until January 1985 that the first DSN was officially appointed in Portsmouth (Cradock, 1991). Prior to this, people with diabetes received their care and education from hospital ward staff or community nurses. The majority of nurses working in diabetes care were employed in the early 1980s after the introduction of the U100 insulin, but did not hold the title of DSN (Felton, 1989). Clients needed to be educated in how to safely calculate their dosages to the new strength insulin. Thus, more nurses needed to be appointed to undertake this education. For this reason, consideration was not given to the nurses' role, qualifications and entry criteria in the diabetes care field once clients were able to safely self-administer their insulin.

Few of the nursing posts in diabetes in the 1980s were referred to as specialist nursing posts. Castledine (1982) in his study identified at this time only five DSNs appointed in England and Wales. However, he found that, although respondents held the title of the specialist nurse, none of them possessed all the key characteristics of the CNS role as cited in the literature. Moreover, a major variation in titles (diabetes liaison nurse, diabetes sister, diabetes nurse), responsibilities, grading, job descriptions, payment, and entry requirements was apparent (Da Costa, 2000). Hence, standardisation and consistency in the role of nurses working in diabetes care at the end of the 1980s were seen as an emergent necessity.

Furthermore, as the number and needs of people with diabetes increased, it was clear that nurses working exclusively in that field had to be more skilful and knowledgeable than general nurses. Therefore, the requirement for nurses to be able to identify and solve many diabetes-related problems led to the development of the role of the DSN. Kinson and Nattrass (1984) anticipated that the appointment of DSN posts would be a slow process in the first years. It would also be unlikely for large numbers of these posts to be established in view of competition for resources. Therefore, DSNs would have to consider carefully how best to use their time and talents in order to prove their worth.

Today, nurses holding the title of DSN work wholly in diabetes care, full or part time, and are based in the hospital or community, but may visit either, depending on the need and their job description and responsibilities. They work either with adults or children with diabetes and their families/carers, or with both. Many DSNs provide an out-of-hours, weekend advisory service. This is very much valued by people with diabetes, as a telephone call for advice may prevent acute situations arising (MacKinnon, 1998a). This community-hospital remit gives the DSN a unique overview of the healthcare context of patients and their families.

According to Padmore (2000), the DSN as an expert clinical nurse of a higher level should not be tied to a department but allowed to move freely within the organisation and beyond. In this way, they become available and accessible to a range of professionals, patients, carers, teachers, employers and many others, as a consultant in the field of diabetes. The role of DSNs and their responsibilities differ from district to district; inevitably, the diabetes nursing service differs from place to place. Furthermore, DSNs are autonomous, yet are members of, and work in, a multidisciplinary diabetes team and with many other teams in primary and secondary care setting (MacKinnon, 1998b).

The number of DSNs has increased rapidly in the past decade. In 1993 there were over 700 in post (British Diabetic Association, 1993) and almost ten years later more than 1,000 DSNs were employed in the UK (Diabetes UK, 2000). However, regardless of the above DSNs numbers, there is still a significant need for further appointments when taking into consideration the rapid increase in the prevalence of diabetes.

1.4.2 Definition of the role of the diabetes nurse specialist

The role of the DSN is difficult to define, as it is interpreted in different ways, according to locality and/or patients' needs and expectations. Some may view the CNS, including the DSN, as medical assistants and not specialists. Bowman and Thompson (1990) argue that, although DSNs have a supportive and educational role, their skills stem from a medical knowledge base. Cradock (1993) views the DSN as a senior nurse who provides expert direct patient care and is able to influence other healthcare professionals providing diabetes care. It is evident that the DSN role has not been clearly defined. The variation in role titles and responsibilities of specialist nurses working in diabetes led to confusion, which had negative consequences to the development and definition of their role.

The general definition of the role of the diabetes specialist nurse (DSN) conforms to that of the CNS, although it considers other significant and exclusive parameters within the diabetes nursing speciality. According to the Royal College of Nursing (1991; p6), the DSN is '...flexible in time and location of work, permanently involved in diabetes care, innovative, and able to liaise with a variety of hospital and community personnel.' DSNs, while practising in the sub-roles constituting the CNS role, differ from the CNS prototype in some important respects. DSNs are not uniformly Master's prepared, although the majority hold postgraduate qualifications in diabetes recognised by the UK Nursing and Midwifery Council (NMC), i.e. the English National Board Course (ENB) 928 or 998 (Crowley, 2000). In addition, compared to CNSs in the USA, DSNs (as with all CNSs in the UK), although required to be registered with the NMC in order to practise, do not have professional certification for their speciality. However, as mentioned earlier, this is expected to change given the implementation of the NHS Knowledge and Skills Framework (Department of Health, 2004).

In order to clarify and offer a definition for the DSN, in 1991 the RCN Diabetes Nursing Forum Working Party published a document which addressed the responsibilities, title, career structure, and required qualifications for the role (RCN, 1991). To date, this is the only formal document to define the role of the DSN in the UK. The Working Party accepted the definition given by Castledine (1989) that the DSN is a nurse clinician with extended knowledge and skills in diabetes management, an educator, counsellor, manager, researcher, communicator and innovator held responsible for his or her actions.

In addition, the members of the Working Party unanimously agreed to add to the DSN role definition, the following points, particular to diabetes nursing as a speciality:

1. 'The DSN works wholly in diabetes care, either full or part time;
2. The DSN works with a consultant physician or paediatrician with an interest or involvement in diabetes care, or with a consultant diabetologist;
3. The DSN is based in the hospital or community, but may visit either, depending on need, regardless of the funding of the post;
4. The DSN works either with adults or children with diabetes, and their respective families, or both;
5. The DSN is a resource and advisor in nursing issues in diabetes for other health professionals in the health authority;
6. The DSN is an educator in diabetes of colleagues in nursing and other disciplines, in hospital and the community; and
7. The DSN works within the diabetes care team working towards a comprehensive and integrated diabetes service to the employing authority' (RCN, 1991; p7).

Despite the attempts made to define the role of the DSN, it is regrettable that the definition still remains debatable and the qualifications, attributes and experience necessary seem to be open to personal interpretation or institutional preferences. There are many

DSNs who are paid at different rates and/or have different educational preparation or experiential background, but are doing ostensibly the same job (Watkinson, 1997). Therefore, it can be concluded that the clarification of the role definition for the DSN, as for all other CNSs in the UK, and the establishment of a commonly agreed general role definition and core description are crucial to successful role implementation.

1.5 Summary

The evolution of the role of the clinical nurse specialist in the USA and the UK, as well as its definition and characteristics, was presented in this chapter. It was concluded that the CNS role in the UK has followed the development pattern of the CNS in the USA. However, further clarification of this role is needed, especially with regards to the CNS educational preparation and certification.

The evolution and definition of the role of the diabetes specialist nurse (DSN) were also presented in this chapter. This role conforms to the general definition of the CNS role in the UK and requires further clarification. A nationwide study was undertaken aiming to explore the role of the DSN in the UK. This is discussed in the following chapters. A theoretical framework derived from role theory underpinned this study; the development of this framework is presented in the next chapter.

2

Role theory in exploring the role of the clinical nurse specialist

2.1 Introduction

The CNS role performance does not exist in isolation, but is influenced either positively or negatively by many factors and/or expectations. The literature regarding the CNS role is very broad and covers a wide variety of concepts, not all related to role performance.

For these reasons, a firm theoretical framework to guide the review of the CNS literature according to the objectives of the study was crucial. This was also necessary to underpin the investigation of the CNS role and the discussion of findings. As the main concept under investigation was that of 'Role', role theory was considered the most suitable means of guiding the exploration of the CNS role.

This chapter explores concepts related to the CNS role derived from role theory. The first part presents the importance of utilising a theoretical framework to guide this study. In the second part, role theory is defined and its importance in the study of roles highlighted. The development and perspectives of the role theory field are also introduced. The concepts relevant to the CNS role are identified, and constructed into a theoretical framework according to their associations with each other. Finally, the concepts that are explored in this book are listed, and hypotheses are made with respect to their associations with each other.

2.2 Rationale for utilisation of a theoretical framework

The utilisation of a theoretical (conceptual) framework in studying the role of the CNS is of vast importance. There seems to be a consensus that research lacking in theoretical soundness is of little practical use in the development of a professional and scientific knowledge base. According to Polit *et al* (2001), the purpose of theory is to make scientific findings meaningful; therefore, linking theory and research is vital to the development of nursing knowledge. Dickoff and James (1968) were two of the first nursing theorists who called for theory-linked research.

According to Fawcett and Downs (1992), the relationship between theory and research is dialectic: theory development relies on research and research relies on theory. Moreover, Polit and Hungler (1999) state that theory and research have reciprocal and beneficial ties, and their relationship has been described by Fawcett (1997) as a double helix. Nursing research serves as an instrument or tool, the purpose of which is inquiry into the development of nursing and the extension of knowledge, with a means to improved patient care. The function of research is either to generate theory through the study of nursing phenomena, or to test the validity of an existing theory (Dickoff *et al*, 1997).

However, in a case where a phenomenon or role has not been previously studied, theory functions as guidance for the research process. McKenna (1997) used the term 'Theory-framed research' (TFR) to describe this type of theory-research linkage, and states that its purpose is to guide the research study, to provide it with focus, and to determine what questions will be addressed by the study and how the data will be collected. The same author notes that when theory is used as a theoretical framework, it:

- 'Gives direction to the investigation;
- Abstracts, summarises and orders research findings;
- Relates the study to previous work' (McKenna, 1997; p206).

The theoretical framework used to guide the research process may be a theory borrowed or adapted from another discipline, a nursing theory or a combination of theories or particular concepts of those theories. According to Brink and Wood (1994), a theoretical framework is simply an explanation, based on the available literature, of how and why different concepts are expected to relate to each other. When some knowledge is available to describe the relationships among the concepts studied, a conceptual framework can be drawn, but it is understood that the relationships diagrammed are tentative and must be confirmed in the empirical phase of the research. Creative appraisal and use of literature is a tool for the development of the theoretical framework (Artinian, 1982).

2.3 Definition and importance of role theory in the study of roles

The theoretical framework underpinning the exploration of the CNS role was devised, based on concepts from the field of role theory. According to Biddle (1979), the field of role theory is of central importance in the study of human behaviour, and the main concern of role theorists is to understand and explain many of the same complex aspects of this behaviour. According to Conway (1988a; p63):

> '*...role theory represents a collection of concepts and a variety of hypothetical formulations that predict how actors will perform in a given role, or under what circumstances certain types of behaviour can be expected.*'

Although a number of schools and perspectives have been developed within this field, authors use the term 'role theory' to refer to the study of individual or group roles and behaviours. However, Thomas and Biddle (1966a; p18) clarify that, although called Role Theory, it is not a grand theory; rather it is a 'field of role' which causes much speculation, and

> '*...consists of many hypotheses and theories concerning particular aspects of its domain, but these propositions, like the knowledge to which they relate, have yet to be reviewed and integrated.*'

Later, Hardy (1978a) agreed with Thomas and Biddle (1966a), stating that it is more accurate to talk about a role framework: the term 'role theory' refers to a selected body of concepts and research with specific orientation towards social structure and social behaviour. In this book, the term 'role theory' is used in accordance with the assertion of

Thomas and Biddle (1966a) that it is not a grand theory, but rather refers to the field of role theories and perspectives.

Role theory has evoked enthusiasm in scientists from different disciplines interested in the study of human behaviour, such as anthropology, sociology, psychology and other health professions. The interdisciplinary nature of role theory offers a meeting ground on which the various social sciences can come together (Biddle, 1979). However, Hardy (1988) pointed out that its interdisciplinary nature and the scientific work that comes from both clinical and academic settings, and the use of its terms by persons who promote different perspectives, not only add to the richness of the conceptualisations but also add to the conceptual confusion.

Role theory concepts are based on common language and appear natural and easy to measure. Moreover, role theory has been commended for the rigour of its empirical research, as its concepts have been studied with a wide variety of research tools, methods and approaches. Furthermore, role theory presents a unique field of study by combining perspective, language, knowledge, theory and research endeavour (Biddle, 1979; Thomas and Biddle, 1966a). For these reasons, health professionals are in a prime position to make use of the role theory concepts and introduce new concepts and ideas respective to the healthcare setting.

2.3.1 The development and perspectives of role theory

The term 'role' as the central idea of role theory and role-related concepts has been cited in the writings of social philosophers, psychologists and anthropologists, such as James, Baldwin, Dewey, Durkheim, Sumner, Cooley and Piaget at the end of the eighteenth century and the beginning of the nineteenth. Although these authors contributed to the development and understanding of role concepts, they did not refer to these concepts in technical or scientific terms (Hardy, 1978a; Riggin, 1982; Thomas and Biddle, 1966a). The systematic study of roles only began in the 1930s, and the role theory field developed rapidly in the period between the early 1960s and middle of the 1980s. The theoretical literature after this period is limited, and the literature in this area is represented mostly by empirical studies.

Among other early theorists, Mead, Linton and Moreno made a significant contribution to role theory development, concept differentiation and refinement. Mead (1934), a social philosopher and originator of the Symbolic Interactionist Role Theory, saw the evolution of roles through reciprocal social interaction and the development of self through the social process, where individuals learn to evaluate themselves as social objects. He introduced Socialisation and Role-taking, concepts that indicate how roles are learned. Symbolic Interaction emphasises the meanings that significant things or symbols have for human beings. These meanings arise from reciprocal interaction and are used by individuals, or modified according to their interpretations of internal and external cues obtained within the process of interaction (Blumer, 1969). Moreover, Symbolic Interaction focuses on individuals and their social integration and embeddedness in a social context, and the reciprocal social processes within which individuals are engaged (Hardy and Hardy, 1988a).

The Structural-Functional Role Theory was first introduced by Linton, an anthropologist. This asserts that roles are linked to structural positions within social context, and consequently, the person is linked to performing multiple roles within the confines of these positions (Hardy and Hardy, 1988a). Linton (1936) perceived 'role' as an external constraint, and associated the behaviour of individuals with the position they occupy in a social system. He was the first to make a distinction between the concepts of Status (position)—a collection of rights and duties, and Role—the dynamic aspect of status. Linton stated that:

> *'The individual is socially assigned to a status and occupies it with relation to other statuses. When he puts the rights and duties which constitute the status into effect, he is performing a role.'*
>
> (Linton, 1936; p114)

Cognitive Role Theory focuses on the relationship between role expectations and behaviour, and the impact of expectations on social conduct. It is also concerned with how persons perceive the expectations of others and how those perceptions influence behaviour (Biddle, 1986). Moreno (1934), a psychiatrist and originator of this approach, worked with psychodrama and introduced the concept of role-playing. His main interest was concentrated on changing human behaviour through role-playing, which may be '...considered as an experimental procedure, a method of learning to perform roles more adequately' (Moreno, 1960; p64).

The fourth perspective, the Organisational Role Theory, originated in the work of Gross *et al* (1958), and was further expanded by the work of Katz and Kahn (1978), and Kahn *et al* (1981). This perspective focuses on the study of roles in formal organisations which

> *'...are assumed to be associated with identified social positions and to be generated by normative expectations, but norms may vary among individuals and may reflect both the official demands of the organisations and the pressures of informal groups.'*
>
> (Biddle, 1986; p73)

Despite the different perspectives of role theory, Conway (1988a; p72) states that none of them '...alone adequately accounts for the wide variety of human responses possible in the numerous and ambiguous situations where human actors confront each other', and recommends the development of conceptual or theoretical frameworks which include concepts from different perspectives. Biddle (1986; p87) views role theory as an inseparable field and suggests

> *'...the gradual evolution of an integrated version of role theory...* [which] *...is likely to explain a lot more about human conduct than current, limited versions of theory.'*

Therefore, it is important that the large and complex domain of role theory is analysed and elucidated. Moreover, the theoretical and empirical knowledge in the field needs to be reviewed, collated, organised, appraised, and formulated into general statements. It is therefore necessary to establish an explanatory theory for the role field (Biddle, 1979; Thomas and Biddle, 1966a).

Although this introduction into its perspectives was deemed necessary, the detailed discussion of a broad and complex field such as role theory goes beyond the purpose of this book. It is sufficient to say that the theoretical framework of this study was based on those concepts of role theory that can be implemented in the exploration of the role of the CNS, and is not biased towards any particular perspective. The following section is concerned with the exploration of role theory concepts that relate to the study of the CNS role and their interrelation within a theoretical framework that underpins the exploration of this role.

2.4 The relevance of role theory concepts to the CNS role

The exploration of the term 'role' in relation to nurses' activities constitutes a significant part of the nursing literature. More specifically, the CNS role has been given great consideration by nursing scholars, although the empirical exploration of this role has focused only on partial aspects of it (Aikin *et al*, 1993; Castledine, 1982; Chambers *et al* 1987; Georgopoulos and Christman, 1970; Hamric and Spross, 1989; McGee and Castledine, 1998; Nuccio *et al*, 1993; Robichaud and Hamric, 1986; Scott, 1997; Sparacino, 2005; Sparacino and Cooper, 1990; Tarsitano *et al*, 1986).

It is evident that role theory concepts can be related to health professions and in particular to nursing (Hardy and Conway, 1988; Hardy and Conway, 1978). Hence, it was felt that the investigation of the integrated role of the CNS should be conducted with reference to role-related concepts derived from role theory that had been previously utilised and validated.

Literature shows that the role of the CNS is influenced by the following factors: personal attributes and motivation; reciprocal interaction with significant others, salient to his/her role; structure of the social environment and employing organisation; and expectations that the CNS and significant others hold for this role. Due to the multifaceted and complex nature of the CNS role, none of the role theory perspectives alone could provide an adequate insight into it; therefore, relevant concepts derived from all perspectives of the role theory field and combined into a theoretical framework were required to explore the CNS role.

Before examining concepts of role theory that relate to the CNS role, it is essential to give a brief description of the meaning of the concept of role as presented within role theory, and related to nursing. One of the constraints of role theory is that the definition of role varies from author to author. The idea of role has been used:

> '*...to denote prescription, description, evaluation, and action; it has referred to covert and overt processes.* [However,] *...perhaps the most common definition is that role is the set of prescriptions defining what the behaviour of a position member should be.*'
>
> (Thomas and Biddle, 1966a; p29)

Role has also been viewed as a set of norms and shared expectations that apply to the incumbent (occupant) of a position and govern his/her behaviour (Banton, 1965; Graen, 1976; Sarbin and Allen, 1968; Scott, 1970). This set of behavioural expectations is formed by *significant others*, whose expectations are particularly salient to the role incumbent (Rosse and Rosse, 1981). For a nurse, significant others may be patient/clients and their families, nurse managers, physicians, colleagues, hospital administrators, or employing organisations. Meleis (1975; p265) suggested that '...role, as a concept, is useful in interpreting personal behaviour vis-à-vis significant others and in understanding the context in which behaviour takes place.' Roles can be ascribed or achieved. When there is no control over the role played, it is said to be ascribed, and includes factors such as age, gender, social class and ethnic origin. Achieved roles are those filled through individual effort and competition, and include educational and occupational levels (Elkin and Handel, 1989; Kelly, 1982). Professional roles are considered to be achieved roles.

Biddle (1979; p56) determined that '...the role concept centres upon behaviours that are characteristic of persons in a context.' This book explores the role behaviour of CNSs in their occupational context. Role theory, as defined by Biddle (1979), is concerned with the study of human behaviours and the factors that influence those behaviours. The CNS role is influenced by expectations that CNSs themselves and significant others hold for this role. Incompatible role expectations lead to role stress and role strain. Moreover, this role is determined by the CNS socialisation into a role; that is, the process in which CNSs acquire the knowledge and skills to perform their role.

On the basis of the above assertions, the exploration of the role theory literature indicated that the following concepts are significant in the study of the CNS role: personal factors (personal characteristics, attributes and skills of the CNS in relation to their role performance); context (the organisational context in which the CNS role performance takes place); role performance; role socialisation (development of role); role expectations; role stress and role strain resulting from incompatibility of role expectations. As can be seen in *Figure 2.1*, depicting the construction of these concepts into a theoretical framework, such concepts have linear reciprocal relationships with one another. They are explored in detail in this chapter.

The design of the theoretical framework was in part influenced by the work of McGarvey (1998), who examined the role of the nurse in the operating theatre department. The theoretical framework that underpinned her study was derived from role theory as defined by Biddle (1979), and constituted three interrelated basic concepts: person, context and role performance. The concepts of role expectations and role socialisation were subsumed within these three basic concepts.

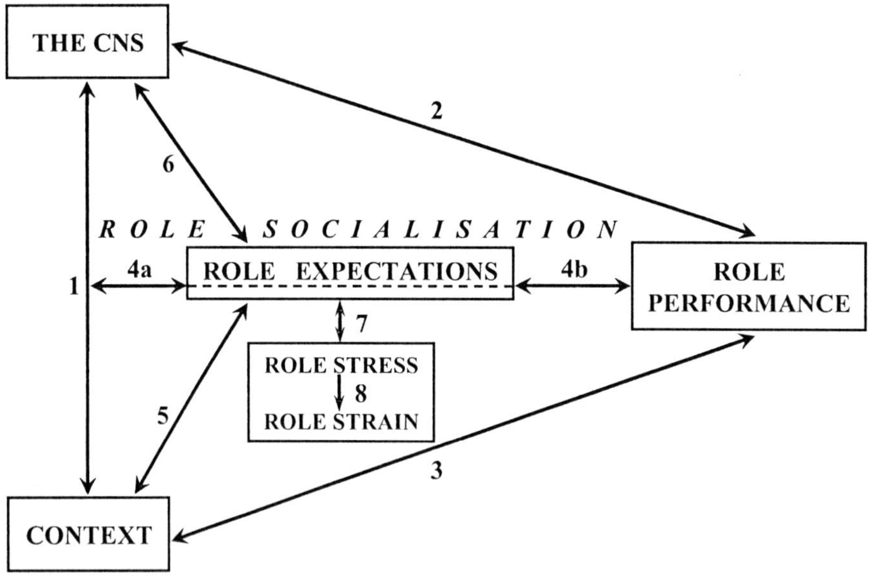

Figure 2.1: Theoretical framework underpinning the exploration of the role of the clinical nurse specialist

To summarise, the relevance of the present theoretical framework to the study of the role of the CNS was supported by the underlying assertions of role theory:

- Behaviours are patterned and are characteristic of persons within contexts (Biddle, 1979). Individuals and their behaviours are dominated and shaped by their social environment, but, in turn, under favourable conditions, they can change and mould social environment (Linton, 1936) [*Arrow 1*]
- Characteristics possessed by individuals, such as attitude, appropriate experience, and specific training, result in effective and convincing role enactment (Sarbin and Allen, 1968). Individuals' values, attitudes, motives and beliefs influence their role performance within the social and organisational environment. Similarly, effective performance increases satisfaction and motivation in enacting the particular role (Katz and Kahn, 1978; Merton, 1968) [*Arrow 2*]
- The incumbent's role performance is influenced by the context and the individuals who perform in this context. On the other hand, adequate role performance can shape the context in which role takes place in response to expectations for this role (Biddle, 1979; Katz and Kahn, 1978) [*Arrow 3*]
- The concept of socialisation explains how role expectations are conveyed and roles are learned (Biddle, 1979). It is a continuous non-ending process by which individuals acquire the knowledge and skills to perform their roles adequately within society (Bandura, 1977; Brim, 1966; Hurley-Wilson, 1988). Almost any normal individual can be trained to perform almost any role adequately (Linton, 1936). The incumbent's socialisation is influenced by a third-party standpoint (context) which indicates what role behaviour is expected from the incumbent (Turner, 1966) [*Arrow 1*; *Arrow 4a–b*]

- Role expectations affect role performance, operate as imperatives pertaining to individuals' conduct and cognition while they enact their roles, and integrate individuals with the social structure. Incumbents and occupants of interdependent positions hold role expectations for each other, and their expectations are determined to a considerable extent by the broader organisational context (Calkin, 1988; Conway, 1988b; Katz and Kahn, 1978; Sarbin and Allen, 1968) [*Arrow 4b*; *Arrow 5*; *Arrow 6*]
- A condition of role stress is identified when role expectations held by the social structure (context) are incompatible with those of its role incumbents and affect both parts. The occurrence of role stress results in impaired role performance (Hardy and Hardy, 1988b) [*Arrow 5*; *Arrow 6*; *Arrow 7*; *Arrow 4b*]
- The role incumbent responds to the occurrence of role stress with role strain, which is the difficulty felt in meeting role requirements (Hardy and Hardy, 1988b) [*Arrow 8*].

The next six sections present a detailed exploration of the concepts that compose the theoretical framework underpinning the exploration of the CNS role. However, although presented separately, they are in fact interrelated and overlap with each other. The following concepts are discussed with reference to nurses' roles in general and to the CNS role in particular. Reference is also made to the role of the diabetes specialist nurse (DSN) as the empirical exploration of these concepts involved DSNs.

- Personal characteristics (the CNS)
- Context for role performance
- Role expectations
- Role stress and role strain
- Socialisation into role
- Role performance.

2.4.1 Personal characteristics

According to Biddle (1979), roles are performed by persons, and the concept of role is confined to the behaviours of human beings. Therefore, to some extent, incumbents' individual characteristics and personality shape their role performance. Individuals differ in intelligence, temperament, and in the learning that they have acquired. Those differences can be reflected in their particular total behavioural repertoire (Thomas and Biddle, 1966b). Brim (1960) stated that, in order to conform to the demands of the role they perform, individuals must:

1. Know what is expected of them in a situation (adequate knowledge of a role);
2. Have the ability to fulfil the demands of a role upon them; and
3. Be motivated to perform a role.

The above variables describe the learning that individuals have accrued regarding a role, and thus the level of their socialisation into that role (described later in this chapter).

The individual is ascribed a set of positions and roles, such as age, gender, and ethnic origin, and the remainder are hypothetically open for membership (achieved roles). The individual is responsible for choosing among behavioural possibilities (Biddle, 1979). However, according to Thomas and Biddle (1966b), not all the open positions or roles are viable alternatives and the individual's choices will be determined by various factors. Some roles are culturally disapproved and some too difficult to enter, or demand relatively high achievement. Furthermore, individuals face a particular environment of others who hold expectations of, and make demands upon, them, describe their behaviour in given ways and react to them with approval or disapproval. Therefore, the choice of a role does not depend entirely upon the incumbent. As early as the 1930s, Linton (1936; pp95–96) posited that individuals' behaviour is affected by their society, but he also pointed out that:

> *'Although the individual is dominated and shaped by his social environment, he is not obliterated by it. Under favourable conditions he can even change and mould it. Thus the personality of an outstanding individual, such as a successful religious leader, may leave a mark upon his society which will endure for generations.'*

The outstanding personality of Florence Nightingale gave the light for the development of nursing as a science and marked its history. It can be asserted, therefore, that persons are mutually affected by their social environment (context) and their roles are performed through continuous reciprocal interaction with this.

With regard to occupational roles, role incumbents are selected according to the personal characteristics they must possess in order to perform their roles efficiently. Moreover, role expectations are influenced and/or modified by the characteristics of the incumbent (McGarvey, 1998; Topham, 1987). In this case therefore, '...a "person" is simply a human being who is related to task elements through a co-ordinating set of relationships called a position' (Oeser and Harary, 1966; p93). How well individuals will perform these tasks, besides variables such as role expectations, context, and role demands, depends on their differential role skills. According to Sarbin and Allen (1968; p514), these are:

> *'...those characteristics possessed by the individual which result in effective and convincing role enactment: attitude, appropriate experience, and specific training. ...Persons differ in basic attributes, in past experience, and in relevant training, all of which interact to influence role enactment* [role performance].'

Role skills are not inherited; they can be acquired through the process of socialisation and the individual's role-learning abilities. According to Linton (1936), almost any normal individual can be trained to perform almost any role adequately. An adequate educational preparation of nursing students in the area of personal and professional socialisation increases students' ability to cope with the transition from the classroom to the service area (Kelly, 1982). In addition, continuous and appropriate training will enhance the status of their roles and, as Biddle (1979; p70) stated, '...not only will they [roles] be differentiated more clearly from other roles, but also their practitioners will come to be positionally designated and differentiated from others.'

Role theorists, also noted that experience plays an important part in the adequacy of performance of a role. The longer the experience of performing a role, the more adequately the role is performed. Experience, however, as Benner (2001; p36) notes, does not merely refer to the passage of time or longevity, but to '...the refinement of preconceived notions and theory through encounters with many actual practical situations that add nuances or shades of differences to theory.'

Individuals' personal beliefs in, and motivation for, roles are also believed to be related to the adequacy of their role performance. The same role can be viewed and experienced differently by different people, depending on how they perceive, and what they expect from, their role. According to Katz and Kahn (1978), individuals have an occupational self-identity and are motivated to behave in ways that affirm and enhance their valued attributes. However, they further stated that individuals may come to a job in a 'role-readiness' state, which includes the acceptance of legitimate authority and compliance with its requests. This compliance for many people may extend to acts they do not understand or that violate their own values. Cases have been reported where nurses have to undertake actions that are required by the health organisation or the medical profession, although these requirements conflict with nurses' beliefs.

Motivation, as another personal characteristic, refers to what drives role occupants to do what they do (Turner, 1991). According to Conway (1988b), a modern health organisation considers the motivation of its workers to optimal effort in the performance of their jobs to be a very important issue. Moreover, the same author pointed out that highly motivated individual workers produce collectively a high output for the organisation.

It can be seen that there are assertions that incumbents' personal characteristics affect their role performance. However, although these influence their role performance and role expectations, role performance also affects incumbents' personality—people become what they do (Katz and Kahn, 1978). According to Kahn *et al* (1981), the nature of an individual's experience in a role can result to changes in personal attributes, although such changes in personality take place over relatively long periods of time. As Colomy and Rhoades (1983) stressed, personality needs lead an incumbent to adopt a particular, characteristic manner in meeting role requirements, or to develop a particular personal pattern of compliance.

2.4.2 Context for role performance

According to Biddle (1979), roles are limited by contextual specification and do not represent the total set of all behaviours exhibited by the individuals studied at work and at home, 24 hours a day, for 365 days a year. Context is defined as '...any condition or state of affairs that affects behaviour' (Biddle, 1979; p52). Katz and Kahn (1978) relate role to context, and state that the role episode is shaped by contextual factors—individual, interpersonal, and organisational. The organisational context determines to a considerable extent the role expectations held by its members, and, consequently, the role performance of incumbents. In terms of expectations, in a particular setting, the role behaviour of role occupants is influenced by the expectations of others for incumbents' roles. CNSs work in a multidisciplinary team and with many other teams in hospital and community settings (MacKinnon, 1998a). Their role performance is, therefore, influenced by the expectations of other members of the team.

According to Turner (1991), a social organisation is composed of various networks of statuses and expectations. Properties of an organisation, such as technology, structures of its subsystems, its formal policies, and its rewards and penalties, indicate what the role occupant is supposed to do, with and for whom. Moreover, McGarvey (1998) points out that, besides the contextual variables, administrators exercise an indirect effect on the roles of nurses through decisions about the choice of products, technology, and formal division of labour.

Biddle (1979) considers human beings as a type of environmental unit, and states that persons form part of the context within which roles are performed. In an organisational context, according to Kahn *et al* (1981; p167), '...the relative positions of any two persons within this total structure determine to a considerable degree the relations which will obtain between them.' Therefore, the interpersonal relationships between role occupants of an organisational group influence their role performance. However, as Kahn *et al* (1981) pointed out, although the relations between members of an organisational group are considered interpersonal, they are in fact 'largely depersonalised'. The relations between individuals are shaped primarily by the formal structures of organisations, hence positional, rather than personal, attributes become the principal units of analysis. For example, in a multidisciplinary team, the position of each member of the team determines their behaviours and expectations towards other members.

Most of the positional roles are context dependent, indicating that they are important and may change radically from context to context (Biddle, 1979). A CNS performs different roles in different contextual settings. For instance, when she provides education, she acts as an educator; when undertaking research, she acts as a researcher; in her personal life she might be a wife and mother. Thus, researchers who study occupational roles need to confine their attention to observing behaviours in contexts wherein the individual is recognised as an occupant of the position (Biddle, 1979).

2.4.3 Role expectations

Roles never exist in isolation. The role occupants and those around them have notions about what behavioural patterns should be (Holle and Blatchley, 1989). Designated role expectations are the prescriptions and proscriptions held by incumbents and significant other individuals or groups (Katz and Kahn, 1978). Sarbin and Allen (1968; p498) define role expectations as:

> *'...collections of cognitions—beliefs, subjective probabilities, and elements of knowledge—which specify in relation to complementary roles the rights and duties, the appropriate conduct, for persons occupying a particular position. The structure of role expectations is organised in such a way that meaningful behavioural units ("husband", "father", "teacher") are created from what would otherwise be a series of disparate, isolated, and disconnected elements of behaviour.'*

Katz and Kahn (1978) view role expectations being determined to a considerable extent by the broader organisational context. The role expectation of a nurse is shaped by the technology of the organisation, its organisational structure, its formal policies, and its rewards and punishments (McGarvey, 1998). Role expectations act as evaluative standards applied to an incumbent of a position; that is, they evaluate and influence the incumbent's role performance (Gross *et al*, 1958). Moreover, the role incumbent not only endorses behavioural expectations for him(her)self, but also holds expectations for those individuals occupying counter-positions (Jackson, 1998a).

Gerrish (1990) examined the role of the ward sister from a role theory approach and identified a particular body of expectations held for this role. These differed between individuals or groups of people; for instance, patients, other nurses, medical staff, visitors or organisational administration. By attempting to meet these complex role demands, the ward sister may experience role stress and role strain when the expectations are unclear, too many or mutually contradictory.

The concept of legitimacy, as described by Katz and Kahn (1978), is an important attribute of an organisation. Members of the organisation comply voluntarily with the rules and policies of the work setting because they perceive that it is the appropriate thing to do when, in their opinion, the authority of those who make the rules is properly vested (Conway, 1988b).

According to Parker (1997), the standards of care expected from the specialist nurse are those of the competent nurse undertaking those roles. Therefore, as Parker suggests, protocols can be helpful when justifying a nurse's practice. They provide documentary evidence of the agreement between employer and nurse (expectations of the two groups), and define roles and responsibilities. For instance, according to the Code of Professional Conduct (United Kingdom Central Council, 1992b), nurses are required to decline tasks or responsibilities unless they are able to carry them out in a safe and skilled manner. The person who fails utterly to conform to the expectations of role is confronted with removal from their position (Katz and Kahn, 1978). Thus, the inability of a nurse to comply with the regulations set by the Nursing and Midwifery Council (NMC) [known until March 2002 as the United Kingdom Central Council (UKCC)] would lead to his or her exclusion from the National Nursing Register and of any rights to practise nursing.

2.4.4 Role stress and role strain

According to Hardy and Hardy (1988b; p159), 'when a social structure creates very difficult, conflicting, or impossible demands for occupants of positions within it, the general condition can be identified as one of role stress.' Role stress affects both the role incumbent and occupants of interdependent positions, and is mainly external to the incumbent. Social structures, as a vital part of the incumbent's environment, may address incompatible expectations, attitudes, beliefs, and behaviours assigned to an incumbent's social position or set of statuses. Role stress may also result from interpersonal or intrapersonal sources, the location of the role in the social structure, the inadequate resources of role incumbents, and the social context (Hardy, 1978b).

Role stress may generate role strain, which is defined as the difficulty felt in meeting one's role obligations. Role stress differs from role strain in that it refers to conditions generated from impossible, contradictory, incompatible, or excessive role expectations, while role strain refers to the incumbent's reaction to those conditions (Hardy and Hardy, 1988b). Therefore, role stress is a prerequisite for role strain, and they hold a linear relationship; the greater the number of stressors that incumbents are exposed to, the greater the role strain they experience. Halsey (1978) explored the role of the nurse holding a leadership position, and noted that the nurse leader must deal with role prescriptions from a variety of sources. Often the role demands and expectations of one group of people are inconsistent with those of other groups. The nurse leader, when unable to assimilate those conflicting expectations, experiences role strain.

Prolonged role strain places a considerable burden on the person. As Hardy and Hardy (1988b) suggested, if uncorrected, it may have various psychological and physiological consequences on the incumbent, such as anxiety, tension, irritation, resentment and depression. Like role stress, role strain influences both role occupants and occupants of counter positions, and in high levels it disrupts social interaction and prevents goal attainment. In health professions, role strain not only leads to reduced quality of care, but may even jeopardise lives. Moreover, healthcare workers may be drained of both energy and commitment to professional values and patient care.

Response to role strain is influenced by resources of the role incumbent and by characteristics of the social structure (Rubin, 1988), which means that different people react with a different level of role strain to a difficult condition. Most of the time, incumbents do not tolerate role strain indefinitely, undertaking actions to deal with it. They may restructure expectations for their role, develop strategies to cope with the difficulties in overcoming role strain, or decrease the level of involvement by keeping role distance. Resigning from the position is another strategy to resolve role strain (Biddle, 1979). Hardy and Hardy (1988b; p159) suggest the following strategies for the management of role strain:

> *'...redefining the role, redefining what is considered "adequate" role performance, re-establishing priorities within a role and among roles, role bargaining with role partners, and reduced interaction with role partners.'*

Empirical research regarding role stress has mainly focused on its types rather than on role stress in general. Hardy and Hardy (1988b; p162) identify seven classes in the typology of role stress and define each of them as follows:

1. Role ambiguity—vagueness, lack of clarity of role expectations;
2. Role conflict—role expectations are incompatible;
3. Role incongruity—self-identity and subjective values are grossly incompatible with role expectations (role transition and poor self-role fit);
4. Role overload—too much expected in time available;
5. Role underload—role expectations are minimal and underutilise abilities of role occupant;
6. Role overqualification—role occupant's motivation, skills, and knowledge far exceed those required; and
7. Role underqualification (role incompetence)—role occupant lacks the necessary resources (commitment, skill, knowledge).

From the above definitions, it can be seen that all types of role stress are directly associated with role expectations, although they originate from various sources. According to Rodgers-Ward (1986), the function of role stress is to produce role strain when normative and/or role expectations within social structure are inconsistent or conflicting. Hence, when role expectations are congruent with incumbents' perceptions and preferences, role stress is minimal or absent. The literature reveals that the most prevalent types of role stress regarding the role of specialist nurses are those of role conflict, role ambiguity, and role overload.

2.4.4.1 Role conflict

Role conflict, which Biddle (1986; p82) defined as '...the concurrent appearance of two or more incompatible expectations for the behaviour of a person', is often present within the nursing profession. According to Riggin (1982), role conflict in nursing occurs when the incumbents' educational preparation is in contradiction with the bureaucratic or administrative constraints that militate against utilisation of the knowledge, skills, values, and expectations that incumbents hold for themselves as professionals.

Sarbin and Allen (1968) identified two types of role conflict: interrole and intrarole conflict. *Interrole conflict* occurs when the incumbent occupies simultaneously two or more roles or positions, and expectations are incompatible for the different roles. The CNS may be at the same time wife and mother, and then undertake a post-graduate course. If expectations held for each of these roles conflict with each other, the CNS will be exposed to interrole conflict and experience role strain. *Intrarole conflict* occurs when two or more role senders hold contradictory expectations for the same person. For instance, members of the multidisciplinary team may expect the CNS to organise educational sessions for patients or undertake home visits and, at the same time the employing organisation expects her to undertake a research project. Being unable to conform to both expectations simultaneously, the CNS is caught in an intrarole conflict.

Role conflict, if uncorrected over a long period, may have a severe impact not only on the incumbent's personality and role performance, but may also result in disturbance of occupants of counter positions. However, in the short term, role conflict is considered to be a very important source of motivation, which leads to social change through '... some sort of undermining of the motivational bases of an established order which includes the provision of motivationally acceptable alternatives' (Parsons, 1966; p276).

2.4.4.2 Role ambiguity

Role ambiguity occurs when there is a lack of clarity of role expectations. When little information is available on expected performance or the normative expectations for the role are vague, ill defined, or unclear, the role incumbent may experience role strain (Hardy and Hardy, 1988b). In other words, the occupant of a particular role is uncertain about what he or she is supposed to do, and/or how to do it (Biddle, 1979; Katz and Kahn, 1978). Loudermilk (1990) in a review article identified the following sources of role ambiguity for CNSs: inadequate socialisation to the role, conflicting role expectations of administrators and staff, inconsistent job descriptions, poorly defined job qualifications, multiple accountability, inconsistent position within the bureaucratic framework, and unclear criteria for evaluation.

Role ambiguity, like role conflict, although detrimental to the incumbent's role performance when prolonged, provides the opportunity for creativity within the role and in role-making. The incumbent, being intolerant of role ambiguity, strives actively for clarity, structure and continuous definition of role (Hardy and Hardy, 1988b; Kahn *et al*, 1981).

2.4.4.3 Role overload

Role overload occurs when role expectations are excessive relative to the time available. Although able to perform each of the role obligations competently, the role occupant is unable to complete all of them within given time limits. At the same time, all the expectations are of equal importance to the performance of a role. The incumbent experiences role strain due to difficulties in deciding which expectations to comply with and which to hold off (Hardy and Hardy, 1988b; Kahn *et al*, 1981). The large caseloads that a CNS may have contribute to the occurrence of role overload. Evidence exists that the increased workload of CNSs results in inadequate performance of all the activities and sub-roles that are expected of them. The sub-roles that are more frequently affected are those of education and research (Cradock, 1999; Crowley, 2000; Johns, 1997).

2.4.5 Socialisation for roles

According to Biddle (1979), most role theorists use the concept of socialisation to explain the appearance of roles. This is the means by which role expectations are conveyed and roles are learned (Muldoon-Mastey and Cole, 1992). McGarvey (1998) refers to socialisation as the process of induction into roles that have special requirements, obligations and status. Such roles require persons to incorporate new knowledge, alter their behaviour and change their definition of self within the social context. Biddle (1979; p282) defines socialisation as:

> *'...changes in the behavioural or conceptual state of the person that follow from an environmental condition and lead to the greater ability of the person to participate in a social system.'*

Socialisation involves two notions: that of accommodation (environment) and that of learning. According to Goode (1966), the content of a role is partly an organisation of norms as applicable to a particular situation. The application of inappropriate norms for the particular role context is one of the reasons that the individual fails in a role obligation. Therefore, as Goode (1966) further noted, the significance of socialisation is that the individual acquires a commitment to the norms of the society and accepts the rightness of applying a particular norm or norms to a specified situation or context.

The student nurse, for example, has to conform to a series of pre-set role expectations and demands during the educational socialisation process. When the new professional enters the work setting, the process changes, and may present difficulties for many individuals. The nurse is faced with the need to make operational the values of the profession in principally bureaucratic settings, which are not always supportive of professional career development (Leddy and Pepper, 1989). Simpson (1979) explored how nursing students become professional nurses, using data from a longitudinal study in the United States. The study examined the occupational socialisation of successive cohorts of students through their education and in the first year of their nursing practice. It was noted that:

> '*...success of socialisation depends on the educational programme of a school, its fit with the professional culture, and the opportunities it provides for students to assimilate professional-role expectations through experiences that occur within professional-role contexts or can be related to such contexts.*'
>
> (Simpson, 1979; p8)

Socialisation entails social learning. Inherent concepts in socialisation are those of role modelling, role taking and role making. Bandura (1977) pointed out that reflexes are the only inborn behaviours. People must learn all other behaviours, either by direct experience or by observation. They can be learned observationally through modelling, which is: '...from observing others one forms an idea of how new behaviours are performed, and on later occasions this coded information serves as a guide for action' (Bandura, 1977; p22).

Role modelling can be illustrated in the socialisation of nursing students, who learn roles by observing 'model' nurses or nursing tutors, and thereafter base the performance of their role on the information obtained through observation. Theoretical knowledge acquired through education equips the student with a critical understanding of what he/she observes. However, it would be arduous, if not hazardous, if student nurses and novice or inexperienced nurses were to undertake nursing activities based exclusively on their accrued theoretical knowledge.

Bandura (1977) identified four processes of observational learning: attention (attraction to and accurate perception of the significance of the modelled behaviour), retention (ability to remember and rehearse the observed behaviour), motor reproduction (ability to carry out the observed behaviour), and motivational processes (people accept observed behaviours that they find self-satisfying and reject the ones they disapprove).

Role taking, which was first articulated by Mead (1934), is another prerequisite to the learning of roles, development of self and participation in social interaction. It refers to the individual's development of the capacity to take the role of the other; that is, the individual anticipates the response of the other to his own behaviour (Hurley-Wilson, 1988). Following this, the role taker plans and performs his/her role by vicariously assuming the role of the other. The concept of role taking, therefore, suggests that individuals learn roles in pairs through reciprocal interaction, and not singly (Meleis, 1975). Biddle (1986) suggests that people who interact regularly or have similar backgrounds have the ability to take one another's roles more accurately than those who do not.

The process of role taking requires the role incumbent to adopt the attitudes of the other person, to see things from his point of view and to predict his behaviour. Since the behaviour of the significant other is the pattern for the incumbent's further behaviour, any lack of role-taking skills has significant effects on his role performance (Sarbin and Allen, 1968). The student and novice nurse's ability to take on the role of other senior nurses or tutors facilitates their professional socialisation into nursing. Role theorists relate the empathetic component of role skills to taking the role of the other. They define empathy as the ability to put oneself in the other's place, to understand his role and judge his expectations accurately (Biddle, 1986; Sarbin and Allen, 1968; Turner, 1966).

The process of role taking may be also influenced by a third-party view, which indicates the behaviour expected of the incumbent, depending upon the inferences made concerning the role of the other. The third party may be a person or group, or may be depersonalised into a norm. The role of the other in this case becomes a datum necessary implementing the third-party directive (Turner, 1966). Having to conform to the expectation the third party, the role-taker adopts from the role of the other only those behaviours that accor the expectations of the third party.

The procedures of undertaking nursing activities have been determined in different pr cols, and thus, nurses are expected to perform their role in accordance with these protocols. S dent nurses, by taking the role of the senior nurse 'model', will learn to perform their role in same way. If the nurse 'model' does not conform to the expectations of his/her role, the stud nurse, being knowledgeable of what is expected in his/her socialisation into that role, will not ad the behaviours of the nurse 'model'.

According to Conway (1988a), role making refers to the process that takes place when modification is consciously entered into. Role taking and role making both involve taking the a tudes of others who are involved in an interaction. However, the difference in role making is structuring of the interaction in such a way as to modify it and, consequently, to make explicit tain aspects of the role. Role expectations and role prescriptions in nursing and health professi cannot be specified in detail, because these roles are dynamic and often require unpredicta activities or behaviours. Therefore, in the role-making process, the initiated behaviour and response pattern are altered or modified (Riggin, 1982).

Brim (1960) viewed socialisation as successful if it prepares individuals to perform a quately the many roles that will be expected of them throughout society in the course of th careers. This requires an increased repertoire of behaviours by individuals in order to respond variety of situational demands of different complexity. The focus thus is upon the variation wit roles rather than between roles. When consistency in the behaviour of individuals in varied sit tions exists, socialisation is considered to be unsuccessful. This means that role incumbents h not been trained to discriminate between different situations or roles. Therefore, they appea respond to similar circumstances in the same way by implementing a pre-determined list of ru and prescriptions.

As Benner (2001) explains, although making organisational rules explicit facilitates co-ordination and implementation of procedures with some degree of quality control, a nurse m not, for instance, follow the written nursing care plan to the letter. If changes in the patient or en ronment condition occur, the care plan will need to be modified accordingly. Therefore, a nu must acquire the skill of situational assessment and adjustment. Moreover, nurses need to adj the performance of a specific role to the individuality of each person. To illustrate this, let us c sider education as one of the sub-roles of the CNS. Although the performed role is education, CNS uses different approaches when educating patients, carers or health professionals, or e when educating patients with the same condition, as each of them differs in their cognitive a physical abilities.

2.4.6 Role performance

Role performance refers to the differentiated behaviour or action of an incumbent relevant to a s cific position within a context (Hardy and Hardy, 1988b). The majority of the issues and conce that have been examined in the previous sections are related to and influence role performan Therefore, the purpose of this section is to bring together the relevant theoretical issues that rel to role performance. Role behaviour and role enactment are cited in the literature as synonym role performance and are used in this book with equal meanings. Katz and Kahn (1978: p1 define role performance as '...the recurring actions of an individual, appropriately interrelated with the repetitive activities of others so as to yield a predictable outcome.' The set of interdependent behaviours comprises a social system or subsystem in which people perform their roles.

In exploring the role theory literature, the following have emerged as fundamental interrelated antecedents to the CNS role performance:

- Socialisation into role
- Role expectations and prescriptions
- Role stress and role strain associated with incompatible or conflicting role expectations
- Personal characteristics of the role incumbent
- Context for role performance (social and organisational structure, interpersonal relationships with significant parties enacting within the work setting).

Role performance represents the result of the socialisation process of an incumbent into a role. The socialisation process entails the learning of different roles (Biddle, 1979) and thus, depending on its success, socialisation has a significant impact on the role performance of individuals. Moreover, a role is never learned or performed perfectly, therefore the socialisation into a role is a non-ending and continuous process, within which persons acquire the knowledge, skills, and dispositions to enact the particular role (Brim, 1966). The conformity of incumbents to expectations held for their role by the social structure (society, employing organisation) and significant other role senders determines to a certain level the adequacy of the socialisation process and hence, role performance (Goode, 1966; Moore, 1969). Moreover, the personal characteristics required of incumbents to perform a role, such as motivation, skills, knowledge, and innovation, are determining factors in the success of socialisation (Bandura, 1977).

Role performance indicates the behaviour of a person given a set of role expectations. It consists of '...all those expectation-related acts that normally validate one's occupancy of a social position' (Allen and van de Vliert, 1984: p7). According to Sarbin and Allen (1968), role expectations affect role performance. Their clarity and consensus determine the degree to which role performance is convincing, proper, and appropriate. Meleis (1975) states that, in order to enact a role, incumbents need to have a clear idea about the sort of role behaviours others expect them to perform, and an awareness of mutual expectations in complementary roles.

When role expectations are unclear and ambiguous, behaviour will be less predictable, resulting in ineffective and dissatisfying social interaction. Conflicting or incompatible role expectations lead to role stress and role strain, which in turn influence either the incumbent's role performance, or his/her personal characteristics. However, role performance does not imply high conformity to role expectations, as it is not a preprogrammed set of activities, but allows for variability according to the characteristics of the person. Role expectations are usually concerned with broad values or the achievement of certain goals. There is a latitude of acceptability, and within this latitude, a variety of ways of reaching these goals will satisfy role expectations (Allen and van de Vliert, 1984), and consequently allow a smooth progression to the adequate performance of a role. Major (2003) developed a role theory framework to help employed parents cope with their children's chronic illness. She described a role negotiation process applied to meet the emotional and medical needs of the ill child as well as to help parents to maintain their physical and mental health and meet the demands of their other roles such as job expectations.

The performance in a particular role is influenced by incumbents' behavioural tendencies, which are primarily determined by their personal attributes. These attributes include personality characteristics, intelligence, ability, knowledge level, communication skills, interpersonal skills, motivation, and prior experiences (Topham, 1987). Individuals who lack sufficient ability in the cognitive, psychomotor, or social areas relevant to the role will not perform it successfully, although their motivation to do so is very strong (Sarbin and Allen, 1968). Formal or informal training is necessary before role performance is considered appropriate and valid by others (Allen and van de Vliert, 1984).

Finally, the structure of the social setting (context) within which a role occurs influences incumbents' performance in the particular role. Contextual factors, as mentioned in the relevant section, can be individual, interpersonal, and organisational. Within an organisation, behaviours of its role incumbents form a social system. Therefore, as Katz and Kahn (1978: p189) assert, the best way to study role performance is '...to identify the relevant social system or subsystem and locate the recurring events that fit together converting some input into an output.' Understanding the nature of systems in healthcare organisations can help health professionals to cope more adequately with problems that may arise as they attempt to perform their role (Conway, 1988b).

The exploration of the CNS role has, to date, mainly focused on the investigation of components and activities that are subsumed within their role. No previous empirical study explored the CNS role performance in relation to other factors that influence this performance, namely, personal characteristics, context, socialisation into role, and role expectations. Therefore, one of the objectives of the study presented in this book was to examine whether factors combined within the CNS role theory framework influence the CNS role performance.

2.5 CNS role-related concepts explored in this book

In this chapter, the rationale for the exploration of the CNS role using a theoretical framework derived from role theory was justified. The purpose of the study presented in the next chapters of this book was to explore the CNS role performance and the factors that influence this performance from the CNS point of view. However, as only CNSs were involved in the study it was not feasible to examine all the concepts constituting the theoretical framework explored in this chapter.

As noted earlier, not only are role expectations determined by role occupants (CNSs in this case), but also by significant other individuals or groups (Katz and Kahn, 1978). Therefore, role expectations can be explored when all the parties relevant to a role are involved in the study. A number of studies have utilised this approach to examine the expectations held for the CNS role (Boucher and Bruce, 1972; Gaines, 1981; Tarsitano *et al*, 1986).

Hardy and Hardy (1988b) stated that role stress and role strain derive from the incompatibility of role expectations, and are difficult to examine separately. Moreover, role strain reflects reactions (feelings) of role occupants to role stress and, for this reason, a qualitative approach would seem more appropriate for their exploration. In the present study, an open-ended question was addressed to respondents aiming to explore their feelings and experiences relating to their role development (see *Chapter 5*). It was anticipated and confirmed that the data obtained would reveal types of role stress arising from constraints in respondents' practice. However, this approach was tentative and did not aim to examine role stress and role strain.

The limited period of time and resources available for this study hindered examination of all the concepts constituting the theoretical framework underpinning the CNS role exploration. The following concepts were explored:

1. The CNS personal characteristics and skills;
2. Work setting and organisational factors related to the CNS role;
3. The CNS socialisation into role (role development); and
4. The CNS role performance (role components and activities).

2.5.1 Hypotheses derived from the theoretical framework

The following hypotheses were tested:

- The CNS role performance is influenced by their personal characteristics and skills, by work setting and organisational factors related to their role, and by the process of their role development
- The CNS role-related parameters explored in this study, role performance, personal characteristics and skills, work setting and organisational factors, and role development, are mutually interrelated.

2.6 Summary

This chapter discussed the importance of utilising a theoretical framework to guide the exploration of the CNS role. This framework was developed from concepts derived from the role theory field and constituted the following interrelated parameters:

1. Personal characteristics and skills of the role occupant;
2. Context for role performance (work setting and organisational factors);
3. Socialisation into role (role development);
4. Role performance (role components);
5. Role expectations; and
6. Role stress and role strain.

The first four parameters are explored in the next four chapters.

3

Qualifications, skills and personal characteristics of the clinical nurse specialist

3.1 Introduction

The theoretical framework derived from role theory to underpin the exploration of the CNS role was presented in the previous chapter. Four concepts of this framework were examined in a nationwide study involving 334 CNSs working in diabetes. The review of the literature in relation to the qualifications, competences and personal characteristics required by CNSs to perform their role adequately is presented in the first part of this chapter. The second part of this chapter discusses the development of the instrument measuring the DSN personal characteristics and skills. The study finding are presented and discussed in the final part.

Exploratory factor analysis was used to test the instrument exploring the following DSN role concepts: personal characteristics and skills, work setting and organisational factors, and role performance. A detailed description of the study design and methods, as well as the results and statistical analysis, is presented with the aim of providing an insight into the development of a validated questionnaire. It also aims to provide a useful guide for future researchers undertaking similar studies. However, study methods and data analysis are presented only briefly in the following chapters.

3.2 Review of the literature

3.2.1 Basic education, further training and qualifications of the CNS

It has been recognised that initial professional education is not enough to respond to today's complex, expanded, and advanced specialist nursing activities. Meeting the needs of patients and their families demands that CNSs adopt multifaceted roles which require further professional education and training (McGee, 1998). However, according to the International Council of Nurses (1992) specific practice requirements are rare, and a wide diversity in CNS qualifications exists not only between different countries, but also within countries. Although in the USA as early as the 1980s, a Master's degree or its equivalent was recommended for CNS practice (American Nurses Association, 1984), in the UK the entry requirements are still vague and vary from practice to practice. The present requirement for specialist practice is educational preparation at first-degree level (United Kingdom Central Council, 1998), although a Master's level of education is recommended by the latest NHS Knowledge and Skills Framework (Department of Health, 2004).

Graduate programmes for CNS preparation, although divided into specific specialities, should address the common key components of theory content, clinical practice, and research. They should prepare the CNS '...to think critically and abstractly, to assess care situations at an advanced level, and to use and integrate research into clinical practice' (Sparacino, 2005: p419). During the postgraduate educational programmes, CNSs learn to practise the integration of expert clinical judgement, management, education, and consultation skills within their role (Sparacino, 1990). However, a new Master's degree graduate CNS cannot be expected to have expertise in each of the role components. The graduate education provides the CNS with the academic preparation and sets the scientific foundations of role components. Development of expert skills in all aspects of the role must come with experience in the practice setting following graduation.

3.2.1.1 Educational preparation of the diabetes specialist nurse in the UK

DSNs, like other CNSs in the UK, are not uniformly prepared at Master's level of education. However, the majority hold postgraduate qualifications in diabetes recognised by the UK Nursing and Midwifery Council (NMC), such as the English National Board Course (ENB) 928 or 998 (Crowley, 2000).

The Royal College of Nursing (1991) had recommended that, by 1995, newly appointed DSNs would either hold the ENB-928 course on diabetes nursing, teaching and counselling certificates, or would be willing to undertake further diabetes specialist or related courses as in-service development. However, a decade later, there is no evidence to show that these recommendations have been acted upon in all practices in the UK.

The first course designed for nurses caring for the patient with diabetes was established by Janet Kinson in 1978 at the Birmingham General Hospital. Later, the Joint Board of Clinical Nursing Studies in conjunction with Diabetes UK (known then as the British Diabetic Association) approved this course, which is presently known as the English National Board (ENB)-928 Course in Diabetes Nursing Care. The ENB-928 is a 20-day course giving a broad overview of diabetes care designed to teach new developments in this field. Moreover, it gives the registered nurse the opportunity to learn and re-learn the medical, practical, educational and psychosocial aspects of the care of people with diabetes (Cradock, 1991). Today, this course is delivered by a considerable number of universities and diabetes centres across the UK, thus decreasing substantially the accessibility constraints.

Crowley (2000), however, in her study aiming to identify the philosophy, accreditation, content and assessment of available courses on diabetes nursing in the UK, reported variation and lack of standardisation in the ENB-928 courses. Of the 37 respondent institutions that delivered the ENB-928, only seven met the criteria set by the English National Board for a 20-day course involving clinical visits and/or attachments. Crowley found that a significant percentage of the ENB-928 courses were offered within eight to fifteen days and required no clinical placement. Winocour *et al* (2002) collected information on the DSN workforce issues and their grading and training from 351 consultant diabetologists across 238 NHS trusts/units in the UK. Although it was not possible to identify the DSNs' actual educational level, a job specification for this role was recorded in 86% of responses where almost all of them stated that DSNs should hold an ENB-928 or an ENB-998 (course in teaching and assessment).

Nevertheless, even with a length of 20 days, the ENB-928, although essential for the newly appointed DSN, is not appropriate for the further education of a clinical nurse specialist. At present only a small number of universities offer degree and/or postgraduate courses in diabetes (Crowley, 2000). Often those courses present great difficulties of accessibility and flexibility for DSNs who live or work at long distances from the place where they are delivered.

DSNs, as with all CNSs, should undertake postgraduate training that covers all other areas of their complex and broad role besides that of a practitioner; i.e. training in research, education, counselling, and management. Therefore, there is a need for advanced postgraduate courses, which do not have to be solely designed for DSNs, but should include modules to meet the multifaceted needs of the CNS role.

In addition, it is important that not only are expert DSNs highly qualified, but they should also have a pivotal role in the development and delivery of educational programmes that further influence their practice. Crowley (2000) reported that DSNs identified increased workload, limited available time and lack of support as obstacles to their involvement in the delivery of formal education. Many DSNs felt inadequately trained to teach at degree or graduate level, while others reported that universities failed to involve them in the development and/or delivery of academic courses.

It is vital that the practical and experiential knowledge of diabetes nursing is passed on to graduate students by DSNs with expertise in clinical practice. This type of knowledge is non-existent or out of date for tutors who have had limited clinical experience or have never practised as DSNs. Experienced DSNs who are engaged in clinical practice have the ability to share with future DSNs the nuances and complexity of everyday life that can hardly ever be learned through books (Watkinson, 2000a).

3.2.2 The importance of experience in adequate role performance

Experience plays an important part in the adequacy of the performance of a role. The longer the experience in a role, the more adequately the role is performed. According to Benner (2001), clinical expertise is highly influenced by experience with similar patient populations. Expert nurses, with a comprehensive background of experience, have an intuitive grasp of each situation. They no longer rely on analytic principles (rules, guidelines, maxims) to connect their understanding of the situation to an appropriate action. Expert nurses utilise analytic problem-solving methods only when faced with a new situation or when the initial grasp of the problem proves to be incorrect. The nurse who has not seen a range of deviations from normal, although having a theoretical knowledge of the condition, has difficulties in recognising them and in teaching the patient what to expect.

However, this is not the case for the experienced CNS, who gains flexibility and wisdom from working with patients with similar problems, throughout all phases of their condition. The CNS utilises the experientially acquired expertise to develop protocols that may be used as the basis for the care of other patients with the same or similar nursing diagnoses. MacKinnon (1998b) highlighted the importance of clinical experience by stating that only through contact with sufferers of diabetes, allied with the experience gained over time, will DSNs acquire the 'something special' that makes them a 'diabetes specialist nurse'.

Experience, however, as Benner (2001: p178) noted, does not necessarily reflect the length of time or longevity in a position. Rather, it refers to '... a very active process of refining and changing preconceived theories, notions, and ideas when confronted with actual situations.' Practical situations are far more complex than can be described in books, as there is always more to a situation than a theory predicts. Therefore, only concrete experience can provide learning about exceptions in various situations. Theoretical knowledge, however, provides safe and efficient access to clinical learning for the practitioner. It also provides background knowledge that enables the clinician to ask the right questions and look for the correct solutions to a particular problem.

Watkinson (1997) believes that it is essential for DSNs to have at least one year's experience in diabetes care prior to their appointment. She suggested that nurses who wish to develop their career towards diabetes speciality, yet do not have the relevant experience, may join the diabetes team, but should not be given the title of DSN. Clinical experience in the area of interest ideally should start before the CNS enters the post-registration graduate education. The course offers the CNS the opportunity to combine prior experience with theory, and to apply these in practice. In the USA, one of the criteria for admission into a number of graduate speciality programmes has been that applicants must have one to three years of clinical practice in that area (Snyder, 1989).

3.2.3 Personal attributes and competencies of the CNS

3.2.3.1 Personal attributes

The recommended education for a nurse to enter a nursing speciality is at Master's level, but it can be argued that the qualities of the individual are as important as qualifications in becoming an expert practitioner. Those practitioners working in a particular area who are creative, articulate, assertive, visionary, and able to push the confines of practice to conceive new and innovative ways of delivering nursing care are specialist or advanced practitioners.

Patterson and Haddad (1992) referred to attributes and characteristics which identify an advanced practitioner. These include: risk taking (trying out new ideas), vision (utilising and evaluating nursing research to guide patient care), flexibility, articulateness (articulating and disseminating nursing knowledge by formal and informal methods), inquiring mind (participating in nursing research) self-confidence and leadership skills (demonstrating the use of theory-based practice to other nurses).

In a study by Hamric and Taylor (1989: p69), CNSs reported that their personal attributes and skills played a significant part in the successful development and implementation of their role. These included: clinical competence, self-confidence, a sense of humour, motivation, flexibility, interpersonal skills and 'a stubborn streak that would not allow failure.' The ability to listen to the concerns of others and the importance of interpersonal skills has been emphasised, as CNSs have to deal with different types of personalities in their practice (Fenton, 1985; McCaffrey-Boyle, 1997). Moreover, Davis (1994) asserted that CNSs should be able to practise independently and to function autonomously in order to achieve an integrated implementation of their role.

Are there really many CNSs with such inherited talents and qualities? How can administrators assess these attributes when CNSs apply for a job or even after their appointment? With that in mind, why not consider all practitioners working in a specific area or speciality as CNSs, regardless of their qualifications? These questions emphasise the importance of advanced educational preparation for the CNS in order to undertake clinical specialist nursing roles and cope with the requirements of the role. It is recognised that there are currently many capable, knowledgeable and experienced CNSs who do not posses postgraduate academic qualifications. However, with the increasing emphasis on academic and clinical credibility, and as specialist practice requires '...higher levels of judgement, discretion and decision-making in clinical care' (UKCC, 1998: p1), it is imperative that all CNSs are prepared at Master's level.

3.2.3.2 Skills and competencies

Competence in practice is based on set standards, using the identified criteria of professional competency. Therefore, an agreed set of competencies needs to be developed that relates qualifications and individuals' ability to perform tasks at a given level. Confusion exists about the concept of competence, as it involves not only behaviour which can be measured, but also attributes such as attitudes, values, judgemental abilities and personal dispositions, which present great difficulties in their evaluation. Moreover, self-esteem, anxiety and stress, academic experiences, demographic characteristics and availability of good role models can affect the competence levels. A capable practitioner, therefore, is someone who is able to draw on a broad repertoire of skills and knowledge, in different ways and in different contexts, and to perform in a way that is recognised as competent (Lillyman, 1998).

Masterson and Mitchell (2003) presented three types of competence models:

- Personal competence model
- Educational competence model
- Performance outcome model.

Each model has different purpose but can be used in combination to enhance the CNS role performance. The personal competence model focuses on individuals' personal qualities, skills, motives and aspirations that are thought to have a direct impact on role performance. Personal competence concepts, as noted in the previous section, are the distinguishing features of an expert nurse. However, they are often difficult to measure and assess. The educational competence model focuses on what an individual needs to know and be able to do by the end of the learning period. Finally, the performance outcome model focuses on the standards and criteria that the individual undertaking a particular role is expected to achieve.

Practitioners who enter the nursing profession have undergone a process of education and assessment, and are recognised as having attained an agreed level of competence at which they continue to perform. Following registration, practitioners are required to continue to demonstrate that the level of competence has not only been maintained but has also been improved (Lillyman, 1998). CNSs, as practitioners performing at an advanced level of practice, have an obligation to achieve a higher level of competence by maintaining and developing their practice (United Kingdom Central Council, 1990).

The list of competencies suggested as necessary for CNSs is very broad. Snyder (1989) referred to seven significant areas of the CNS skills, which can be further strengthened in a Master's course: leadership and management skills, group process skills, organisational skills, ability to negotiate and debate, ability to develop a support system for oneself, and self-confidence. Fenton (1985) referred not only to the importance of the ability of CNSs to develop their own support systems, but also to the ability to generate their own job satisfaction in order to implement their role successfully. CNSs take responsibility for their own job satisfaction and actively plan to do so without expecting the job or system to supply it.

Other characteristics of CNSs that lead to success are perseverance in their efforts to effect change by acknowledging the fact that immediate change should not be expected. They should also be able to tolerate any ambiguities or constraints of the system. Critical thinking and analysis, clinical judgement, decision-making ability, problem-solving skills, and communication and collaboration skills are also essential for advanced nursing practice (Davies and Hughes, 1995). Furthermore, the ability to institute and effect change in order to improve patient care, particularly through utilising research findings, is a key component of the CNS.

3.3 Design and methods

3.3.1 Questionnaire design

A quantitative approach, utilising a postal questionnaire, was adopted in this study to explore the role performance of the DSN in the UK and the factors that influence this performance. When a postal questionnaire is being designed, it is important that questions are clear and easy to understand, as there is no one to explain their meaning to respondents (Kumar, 1996). The questionnaire utilised in the present study combined five sections, four of which were designed to measure the concepts set out in the theoretical framework underpinning the study. The final section elicited demographic characteristics and academic qualifications of respondents. The questionnaire used in this study is included in Appendix A. The questionnaire explored in this chapter was designed to measure the personal characteristics and skills of the CNS and to determine how these affect their role performance.

In the previous chapter it was asserted that an individual's performance within a role, besides variables such as socialisation (role development), context and expectations, depends on his or her differential role skills. Characteristics such as attitude, appropriate experience, and specific training possessed by the individual result in effective and convincing role enactment (Sarbin and Allen, 1968). Therefore, this section aimed to identify and to explore the personal characteristics, attitudes and skills of the DSNs, as well as to determine whether their role performance is influenced by these parameters. The literature review revealed rich information regarding the personal characteristics and attitudes of specialist nurses related to their role. However, no relevant instrument or scale previously tested was identified which could be adopted to explore the DSN role. For this reason, this section of the questionnaire was designed based on the information derived from the literature.

According to Loewenthal (2001), when a questionnaire is being designed, it is very important to choose the appropriate format for eliciting responses. Likert scaling has been widely used in instruments measuring opinions, attitudes and beliefs. Items in a

Questionnaires were sent to 670 DSNs working in the following ten NHS Executive regions of Great Britain: Eastern, London, North West, Scotland, Northern and Yorkshire, South East, South West, Trent, Wales, and West Midlands. The return of the questionnaire indicated consent to participating in this study. Seventeen questionnaires were returned because the participants (all female) had changed address, giving a final sample of 653 DSNs: 628 female and 25 male.

3.3.4 Data analysis

The 334 returned questionnaires contained valid data and were included in the analysis. The first step in the analysis was to code the responses into numerical data (variables) and enter them into the statistical package used for the analysis and presentation of results. The Statistical Package for Social Sciences—Version 9.0 (SPSS-V9.0) for Windows computer program was used for this purpose.

For the purpose of data analysis, the negatively worded items were reversed when data were edited in the SPSS-V9.0; i.e., 1 (strongly disagree) was edited as 5 (strongly agree), 2 (disagree) was edited as 4 (agree), and vice versa. Descriptive statistics, tables and graphs were used to analyse and present the frequencies of responses. Moreover, Pearson's product-moment correlation test was used to identify any relationships between different variables.

Exploratory factor analysis was used to explore the underlying dimensions (factors) of the items comprising the Personal Characteristics and Skills scale. Although a number of factor-analyses methods can be adopted to determine factors that best represent the interrelations among the set of variables, maximum likelihood exploratory factor analysis was utilised in this study. The advantage of this method, as Kline (1994) asserted, is that it has statistical tests for the significance of the extracted factors. It also maximises the canonical correlations between the variables and the factors. Each factor, in turn, explains the maximum variance in the population correlation matrix, as estimated from the sample correlation matrix. Therefore, maximum likelihood factor analysis, as a method of condensation, has the ability to use sample data to predict the results in a wider population, i.e., inferences are made from sample to population (Kline, 1994; Nunnally and Bernstein, 1994). Since the present study aimed at a generalisation of the findings in the wider context of DSNs, as well as that of CNSs, this method was deemed the most appropriate.

3.4 Results

3.4.1 Demographic characteristics

The overall number of questionnaires returned was 341 (52.2%), of which seven were incomplete, and therefore not usable, giving a final response rate of 51.2% (334 DSNs). *Table 3.1* presents the sample of participants and the number of DSNs who returned the questionnaires for each NHS Executive Region of Britain respectively.

Table 3.1 Sample of participants and respondents in the study working in all NHS executive regions of Britain

NHS Executive Region of Great Britain		Sample of participants		Sample of respondents	
		Count	%	Count	%
1.	Eastern	45	6.7	26	7.8
2.	London	74	11.3	22	6.6
3.	North West	86	13.2	39	11.7
4.	Scotland	68	10.4	36	10.8
5.	Northern and Yorkshire	78	11.9	46	13.8
6.	South East	78	11.9	46	13.8
7.	South West	59	9.0	45	13.5
8.	Trent	59	9.0	27	8.1
9.	Wales	42	6.4	22	6.6
10.	West Midlands	64	9.8	25	7.5
	Total	653	100	334	100

Eighty-nine (26.6%) respondents were working part-time as DSNs and 245 (73.4%) full-time. With regard to work setting, 97 (29%) respondents were based in hospital, 43 (12.9%) in the community and 194 (58.1%) were working between hospital and community. The overwhelming percentage of respondents, 325 (97.3%), were qualified as registered general nurses (RGNs). Additionally, 57 (17.1%) respondents were qualified as registered sick children's nurses (RSCNs), 68 (20.4%) as district nurses (DNs), and 48 (14.4%) as registered health visitors (RHVs). Many respondents held more than one qualification.

3.4.2 Educational (academic) qualifications

Forty-four (13.2%) missing values were recorded for the variable 'What is the highest academic qualification you have earned in nursing?'. Of the remaining 290 (86.8%) respondents, the majority (38.6%) held a Degree in Nursing and 7.6% held qualifications such as RGN, RSCN and RHV, identified by the 'Other' category (*Figure 3.1*).

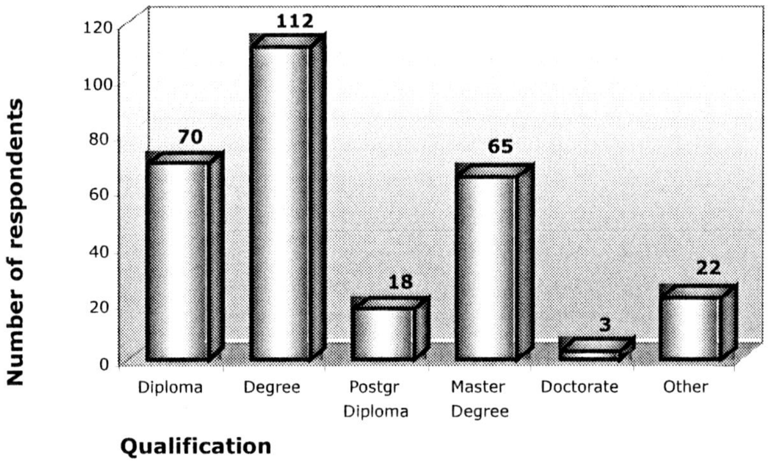

Figure 3.1 Highest qualification in nursing earned by respondents (N=290)

In addition, 264 (79%) respondents had undertaken (or were undertaking at the time of this survey) further education or training related specifically to their role as DSNs. This type of education is presented in *Table 3.2*, where it can be seen that most respondents had undertaken a National Board Course (ENB)-928. Forty-seven (17.8%) DSNs had obtained or were undertaking a Master's degree related to diabetes.

Table 3.2 Respondents' qualifications related specifically to their role as DSNs (N=264)

Academic qualifications	Number of respondents	
	Count	*Percent*
National Board Course (ENB)-928	182	*68.9*
Other National Board Courses	70	*26.5*
Specialist UKCC recordable academic qualification	23	*8.7*
Accredited short course(s) in diabetes	74	*28.0*
Non-accredited short course(s) in diabetes	57	*21.6*
BSc/BA (Hons) in Specialist Practice	37	*14.0*
Diploma in Diabetes Nursing	53	*20.0*
Graduate Certificate in Diabetes	13	*4.9*
Postgraduate Diploma in Diabetes	19	*7.2*
Master's Degree in Diabetes	47	*17.8*
Other academic qualifications in diabetes	30	*11.4*

One hundred and twenty-six (37.7%) respondents had undertaken (or were undertaking) academic qualifications which were not specifically related to diabetes but had contributed (or respondents believed they would contribute) to the integration of their role. Of these, 43 (34.1%) respondents had undertaken an academic course related to teaching, such as a Certificate in Education, an Adult Teaching Certificate, an MA in Education or a Registered Nurse Tutor qualification. Respondents stated that this course had enhanced (or they believed it would enhance) the integration of their role through the improvement of their teaching skills, as education of patients and carers as well as health professionals was a major part of their role.

Twenty (15.9%) respondents had undertaken a course related to counselling. This education had improved their counselling skills and had increased their competence in this component of their role. Moreover, it had helped respondents to understand the psychological issues involved in the care of people with diabetes.

Fourteen (11.1%) respondents had undertaken a management course, such as a leadership course, a health service management course, a Postgraduate Certificate in Leadership and Management or an MA in Management. This training had assisted respondents in dealing with management issues, in evaluating practice and identifying gaps in the service, and had improved their organisational skills in team or staff management, as well as in managing budgets.

Eight (6.3%) respondents had undertaken some course relating to computer technology, which they had found helpful in collating and accessing information quickly and efficiently. Four (3.2%) DSNs had undertaken a course in research methods which had improved their skills in this component of their role. Nineteen (15.1%) respondents considered that their research skills were greatly developed through a Master's degree programme. Moreover, they reported that studying at this level had helped them to understand the wide context of 'care' and nursing and had contributed to their overall competence and confidence. It had also enhanced their skills and abilities to practice at an advanced level. Similar comments were made by twelve (9.5%) respondents who had undertaken a course at degree level. However, although respondents cited the importance of the above qualifications, they further emphasised the continuous update of knowledge by reading and attending study days and conferences. Characteristically, one of them reported:

> *'My educational attainments have not been classified as "diabetes" courses. However, I have applied them to my work and therefore view them as having contributed to my development as a DSN. I am not convinced of the need to do "diabetes" courses specifically in order to grow and develop. However, I am also a very self-directed learner'.*

3.4.3 Personal characteristics and skills

The seventeen items constituting the scale measuring the personal characteristics and skills of the DSN were analysed using exploratory factor analysis. These items and the statements that accord to each of them are presented in *Table 3.3*. Items marked with an asterisk (*) accord to negatively worded statements, and their values were reversed for the purpose of data analysis and presentation. *Table 3.4* presents the frequencies of DSNs' responses for the items included in this scale. It can be seen that most items in this section presented a mean higher than 3.80. This indicates that the majority of respondents rated highly their personal characteristics and skills which, according to the literature, enhance the DSN competence within role.

Table 3.3 Items combining the Personal Characteristics and Skills Scale and the statements that accord to each item

Item number and code	Item statement
Competence before DSN post	I believe I had adequate level of competence in the provision of diabetes care before I entered the DSN post
Further academic education*	I feel I should undertake further education in order to maintain/increase my competence as a DSN
Creativity	I consider myself to be a creative person within my role/job
Competence	I believe I am currently highly competent in the provision of diabetes care
Flexibility	There is a high degree of flexibility in my role
Risk-taking ability*	I am reluctant to try out new ideas within the context of my role/job unless I am sure that they will work
Self-confidence*	Sometimes I have doubts about my abilities to perform sufficiently my role as a DSN
Motivation*	Sometimes I feel that my role/job offers me little motivation or challenge
Interpersonal skills	I believe I have good communication and interpersonal skills
Justify need for change	I am able to defend and justify the need for change within my practice
Listen to others	I believe I listen well to concerns of others
Tolerance*	Any ambiguities or constraints in the system within which I work cause me much anxiety and frustration
Decision-making ability	I am able to make fast decisions within my practice
Finding right solutions*	I have difficulties in finding the right solutions to different problems or situations within my practice
Familiarity with work setting	I am familiar with the organisational structure of my work setting and able to identify who has formal and informal power to influence the system
Negotiating for change*	I have difficulties in negotiating with the administrative authority in favour of improvement in the quality of patient care and my working conditions
Perseverance	I am diligent in my efforts to bring about improvement in my area of practice

* *Negatively worded statements*

Table 3.4 Frequency of respondents' agreement or disagreement with the items of the Personal Characteristics and Skills Scale as rated on the five-point Likert scale (N=334)

No	Item code	1		2		3		4		5		Mean	SD
		Count	%	Count	%	Count	%	Count	%	Count	%		
1	Competence before DSN post	55	*16.5*	173	*51.8*	13	*3.9*	70	*21.0*	23	*6.9*	*2.50*	*1.19*
2	Further academic education*	67	*20.1*	152	*45.5*	23	*6.9*	76	*22.8*	16	*4.8*	*2.47*	*1.18*
3	Creativity	-	-	-	-	24	*7.2*	189	*56.6*	121	*36.2*	*4.29*	*.59*
4	Competence	-	-	17	*5.1*	19	*5.7*	174	*52.1*	124	*37.1*	*4.21*	*.77*
5	Flexibility	-	-	12	*3.6*	12	*3.6*	165	*49.4*	145	*43.4*	*4.33*	*.71*
6	Risk-taking ability*	14	*4.2*	39	*11.7*	30	*9.0*	161	*48.2*	90	*26.9*	*3.82*	*1.08*
7	Self-confidence*	-	-	62	*18.6*	28	*8.4*	147	*44.0*	97	*29.0*	*3.84*	*1.05*
8	Motivation*	11	*3.3*	51	*15.3*	13	*3.9*	140	*41.9*	119	*35.6*	*3.91*	*1.14*
9	Interpersonal skills	-	-	-	-	7	*2.1*	190	*56.9*	137	*41.0*	*4.39*	*.53*
10	Justify need for change	6	*1.8*	26	*7.8*	15	*4.5*	184	*55.1*	103	*30.8*	*4.05*	*.91*
11	Listen to others	-	-	-	-	7	*2.1*	205	*61.4*	122	*36.5*	*4.34*	*.52*
12	Tolerance*	55	*16.5*	152	*45.5*	45	*13.5*	66	*19.8*	16	*4.8*	*2.51*	*1.13*
13	Decision-making ability	-	-	28	*8.4*	25	*7.5*	200	*59.9*	81	*24.3*	*4.00*	*.81*
14	Finding right solutions*	-	-	40	*12.0*	23	*6.9*	206	*61.7*	65	*19.5*	*3.89*	*.86*
15	Familiarity with work setting	6	*1.8*	34	*10.2*	27	*8.1*	198	*59.3*	69	*20.7*	*3.87*	*.92*
16	Negotiating for change*	30	*9.0*	96	*28.7*	31	*9.3*	129	*38.6*	48	*14.4*	*3.21*	*1.25*
17	Perseverance	-	-	-	-	16	*4.8*	216	*64.7*	102	*30.5*	*4.26*	*.54*

1-strongly disagree, **2**-disagree, **3**-uncertain, **4**-agree, **5**-strongly agree

* The values of these items were reversed for the purpose of data analysis. Therefore, the reversed scores are presented in this Table, i. e., 1=5, 2=4, 4=2, 5=1.

3.4.3.1 Exploratory factor analysis for Personal Characteristics and Skills

Nunnally and Bernstein (1994) suggested that two stages in the procedure of an exploratory factor analysis should be followed. On this basis, the number of factors which were extracted by condensing the variance shared among the variables was first defined. Following this, the extracted factors were rotated in order to make them more interpretable.

3.4.3.2 Assessment of suitability of data for factor analysis

The primary step was to assess the suitability of data for factor analysis. The sample in this study (N=334) was higher than 300, a size which has been suggested by Tabachnick and Fidell (1989) as a 'good sample size' for factor analysis and reliably estimated correlations. The determinant was used to test for multicollinearity or singularity which refers to very highly correlated items ($r > 0.8$) and indicates that factor analysis may be inappropriate (Field, 2000). In this section, the determinant was 0.0161, which was greater than the minimum necessary value of 0.00001 (Field, 2000), suggesting that multicollinearity was not a problem for these data. In fact, a closer inspection of Pearson's product-moment correlation matrix revealed the presence of a large number of statistically significant correlations between items ($p < 0.01$), but none exceeded the value of 0.80.

The sampling adequacy in this study was measured with the Kaiser-Meyer-Olkin (KMO) and Bartlett's test of sphericity. The KMO value of 0.776 was greater than the recommended minimum value of 0.5 (Field, 2000), suggesting that patterns of correlations were relatively compact and, therefore, factor analysis would yield distinct and reliable factors. This was also confirmed by the highly significant ($p < 0.001$) Bartlett's test of sphericity. Finally, Cronbach's coefficient alpha test showed that the measure of

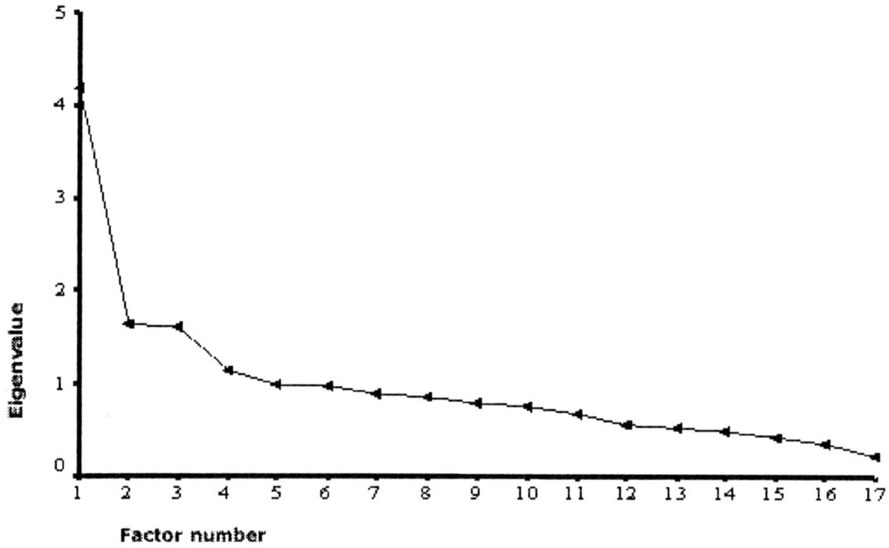

Figure 3.2 Scree plot demonstrating three statistically important factors within the Personal Characteristics and Skills Scale

personal characteristics and skills by the seventeen items of this section was highly reliable ($\alpha = 0.758$).

3.4.3.3 Number of retained factors and their interpretation

Principal components analysis (a method which explains all the variance in a correlation matrix), by utilising Kaiser's eigenvalues and Cattell's scree-plot test techniques, was initially used to identify the exact number of factors to be rotated (Kline, 1994). Kaiser (1960) (cited in Stevens, 1992) recommended retaining all factors with eigenvalues greater than 1. Cattell (1966) (cited in Stevens, 1992), however, suggested retaining the factors in the sharp descent before the first one on the line where eigenvalues start to level off. In the case of non-conformity between solutions obtained from these techniques, the decision is based on the values of communalities. Stevens (1992) suggested that Kaiser's criterion is accurate when the number of items is less than 30, and communalities after extraction are all greater than 0.7. It is also accurate for a sample size larger than 250 and an average communality of all items greater than or equal to 0.6.

In the present study, Kaiser's criterion suggested a four-factor solution. However, the decision was based on Cattell's criterion as only one communality exceeded 0.7 and the mean communality was 0.502. The scree plot depicted in *Figure 3.2* shows that eigenvalues start to level off after the third factor, suggesting a three-factor solution for this scale. After determining the exact number of factors, a maximum likelihood factor analysis with three factors to be extracted was run. To aid in their interpretation, an oblique Promax rotation was selected rather than an orthogonal rotation, because, as reported later in this section, the factors of this scale were correlated.

The three-factor model of this scale explained 33% of the variance: 17% was explained by the first factor, 8% by the second, and 8% by the third. The oblique rotation showed that Factor 1 correlated moderately with Factor 2 ($r = 0.312$; $p < 0.01$) and Factor 3 ($r = 0.384$; $p < 0.01$). However, Factor 2 presented a low correlation with Factor 3 ($r = 0.192$; $p < 0.01$).

The final step in this analysis was to interpret the meaning of the three factors and to determine which items loaded on what factor. Stevens (1992) recommended that for an approximate sample size of 300 a loading equal to or greater than 0.298 can be considered significant. Therefore, any item presenting a lower loading than that was excluded from the scale. Item loadings on each of the three factors of the Personal Characteristics and Skills Scale is presented in a descending order in *Table 3.5*. It can be seen that all factors presented a number of strong loadings and most items loaded substantially on only one factor. However, although items one (competence before DSN post) and two (further academic education) loaded on Factor 1, their loadings are not presented in this table, as they did not exceed 0.298. For this reason, their importance was not considered salient for this model and, therefore, they were excluded from this scale. It should be noted that after excluding these two items, an increase in the internal consistency of this scale was recorded, i.e., Cronbach's coefficient α was 0.775 compared to $\alpha = 0.758$ for the initial seventeen items. Following a thorough examination of the content of the items which loaded on each of the three factors, these factors were interpreted as follows: Factor 1—Competence within Role; Factor 2—Organisational Issues; and Factor 3—Personal Attributes.

3.4.3.3.1 *Factor 1: Competence within Role*

As presented in *Table 3.5*, seven items loaded on this factor. These reflect DSNs' personal characteristics related directly to the degree of their competence within role (refer to *Table 3.3* for a full description of these items). The highest loading (0.896) was recorded for item 4 (competence) which indicates that the greatest percentage (80%) of the variance was accounted for by this factor. In fact, the content and the name itself of this item can justify this result.

When examining items 6 (risk-taking ability) and 70(self-confidence), it can be seen that, although they refer to DSN competence, they also include the attribute of self-confidence; that is, competence is closely associated with self-confidence. The mean score obtained from the scores of items combining this factor indicated that the majority of DSNs reported a high degree of Competence within Role (Mean = 4.0; SD = 0.61). This can also be confirmed by an inspection of the descriptive statistics in *Table 3.4*. Finally, the dimensions of this factor present a highly reliable measurement of this aspect of the DSN Personal Characteristics and Skills ($\alpha = 0.807$).

Table 3.5 Item loadings on each of the three factors of the Personal Characteristics and Skills Scale

Pattern Matrix a

	Factor		
	1	2	3
Item 4: competence	*.896*		
Item 10: justify need for change	*.747*		
Item 5: flexibility	*.655*		
Item 13: decision-makeing	*.554*		
Item 14: finding right solutions	*.517*		
Item 6: risk-taking	*.437*		
Item 7: self-confidence	*.433*		
Item 2: further education	-		
Item 1: competence before DSN post	-		
Item 16: negotiating for change		*.842*	
Item 15: familiarity with work setting		*.548*	
Item 12: tolerance		*.451*	
Item 8: motivation		*.321*	
Item 11: listen to others			*.679*
Item 9: interpersonal skills			*.516*
Item 17: perseverance			*.495*
Item 3: creativity			*.381*

Extraction Method: Maximum likelihood

Rotation Method: Promax with Kaiser Normalisation

[a] 1-Competence within role; 2-Organisational issues; 3-Personal attributes

3.4.3.3.2 Factor 2: Organisational issues

This factor reflected DSNs' ability to deal with different organisational issues and to effect change within their area of practice. This ability was, in turn, influenced by different factors deriving from their work setting. Four items loaded on this factor (*Table 3.5*) (refer to *Table 3.3* for a detailed description of these items). The highest loading (0.842) was recorded for item 16 (negotiating for change) which indicates that the greatest percentage (71%) of the variance is accounted for by this factor. Item 8 (motivation) presented the lowest loading (0.321) on this factor and accounted for only 10% of the variance. This is probably because motivation is both an inherited attribute and it is also influenced by factors deriving from the working environment. Item 8 correlated at a $p < 0.01$ level of significance with other items in the other two factors of this scale—competence within role and personal attributes.

The dimensions of this factor present a moderately lower internal consistency ($\alpha = 0.594$) than those of competence within role. However, considering the low number of items included in this test and the fact that it was tested for the first time, the above value does not necessarily reflect an unreliable measure. Moreover, this factor measures personal characteristics and skills of the DSN and, since personality is a broad construct, lower values of α can be justified.

3.4.3.3.3 *Factor 3: Personal attributes*

The four items that loaded on this factor (*Table 3.5*) refer to personal attributes related to role performance, which are mostly inherited (their detailed description is presented in *Table 3.3*). The percentage of variance which is accounted for by this factor ranged between 15% for item 3 (creativity) with a loading of 0.381 and 46% for item 11 (listen to others) with a loading of 0.679.

The mean score of items combining this factor revealed that the lowest score recorded was 3.50 (Mean = 4.32; SD = 0.37). This indicates that DSNs reported high positive personal attributes relating to their role. In fact, an inspection of the descriptive statistics, presented in *Table 3.4*, shows that more than 90% of respondents reported that these attributes enhanced the performance of their role. As in the previous factor, the dimensions of this factor presented a moderate internal consistency, with a Cronbach's coefficient α of 0.599.

3.5 Discussion

3.5.1 Educational preparation and academic qualifications

It is widely accepted that the basic nursing education is not sufficient for the complex, expanded and advanced practice of a CNS, and that further professional education and training are required. In the present study (39%) of respondents held a degree in nursing and 22% held (or were undertaking at the time of the survey) a Master's degree. Humphris *et al* (1999), in their study of 299 DSNs, found that 18% of respondents held a first degree (BA or BSc) and only 4% held a Master's degree (MA or MSc). It is encouraging to see in this study that a significantly higher percentage of respondents were qualified at both first degree and Master's levels. This indicates the rapid increase in attendance at these courses by DSNs and the importance that a Master's level of education, in particular, is now being given in specialist nursing.

Moreover, when examining the available literature on CNS educational preparation in the UK, it is encouraging to find that DSNs hold the highest qualifications of all groups. The majority of respondents in a nationwide study involving 76 CNSs working in epilepsy had undertaken National Board Course (ENB) courses and 42% held postgraduate qualifications at Diploma level. However, none of the CNSs held a Master's degree (Goodwin *et al*, 2004). Similarly, only 3% of the 657 CNSs working in palliative care were educated at Master's level while 59% held ENB qualifications (Froggatt *et al*, 2001).

The implementation of the Agenda for Change in 2005 in the National Health Service (NHS) aims to evaluate and accredit nursing roles based on a nationally agreed *Knowledge and Skills Framework* (Department of Health, 2004), and recommends Master's level of education for advanced practice nursing.

In the United States, a study undertaken by Scott (1997) showed that all respondents (724 CNSs) were qualified at Master's level. However, a Master's degree was one of the inclusion criteria for participants in this study. Hence, generalisation of findings regarding the educational level cannot be made to the overall population of CNSs working in the USA. According to Sparacino (2000), despite the early recommendations for a minimum qualification at Master's level for CNSs, uniformly accepted standards for educational preparation have not yet been established. A survey of all 50 USA state boards of nursing aiming to clarify preparation for advanced practice nurses was undertaken by Ray and Hardin (1995). Results revealed that in only eleven states did 100% of individuals using the title of CNS hold a Master's degree. Similarly, McFadden and Miller (1994) in their study reported that only 70% of respondents (288 out of 411 CNSs) had been educated to Master's level. However, both studies were undertaken almost a decade ago and latest studies are not available for comparison.

In North America, great emphasis has been placed on the doctoral preparation of CNSs and the continuation of their involvement in clinical practice in recent years (Berger *et al*, 1999; Sterling and McNally, 1999). A study of 20 doctorally prepared advanced practice nurses demonstrated that their active involvement in clinical practice had a great impact on patient outcomes, promoting cost-effective practice and the use of clinical research (Sterling and McNally, 1999). Eighty (12%) CNSs participating in Scott's (1997) study either had obtained or were pursuing doctoral education. Although it is difficult to make cross-cultural comparisons regarding the educational preparation of specialist nurses, only three respondents in the present study were prepared at doctoral level. Similarly, Humphris *et al* (1999) reported that two DSNs held a doctoral degree. Despite this, the fact that doctorally prepared DSNs remain in clinical practice rather than choosing an academic career enhances further the emphasis given during the last years to the advanced educational preparation of specialist nurses in the UK.

In the UK, although a Master's degree is not a requisite, the CNS has to undertake additional educational preparation related to the specific area of specialist practice (Castledine, 1995a). According to Crowley (2000), training and educational programmes are vital to ensure that specialist nurses remain up to date with current changes and integrate these into practice. In the present study, 264 (79%) respondents had undertaken (or were undertaking at the time of this survey) further education or training related specifically to their role as DSNs. The level of these education programmes varied from short courses to Master's degrees.

The results of this study revealed that the majority (69%) of respondents had undertaken a National Board Course (ENB)-928. Similar results were also reported by Humphris *et al* (1999) and Llahana *et al* (2001a). This course was established in 1978, and almost a decade later Redmond (1988) found that 29% of the 123 DSNs involved in her study held an ENB-928. In addition, Redmond (1988) also asked respondents to indicate what they saw as their training needs in the future. It was interesting to find that none of the respondents saw this course as being adequate to meet their future educational needs. Recently, Crowley (2000) found that the ENB-928 was delivered by 37 institutions or universities across the UK, which may be one of the reasons for the high attendance at this course by DSNs. However, a wide variation was found in the curricula, and only seven met the standards set by the National Board of Nursing for a 20-day course that included clinical visits.

With the emphasis now placed on advanced education, and although the ENB-928 and other equivalent courses are essential for the newly appointed DSN, these courses do not meet the broad spectrum of requirements of this role. As early as the 1980s, DSNs perceived the need to undertake a more advanced course than ENB-928 that would lead to a recognised qualification within the specialty (Redmond, 1988). Turner (1987) stated then that courses at graduate level which can foster critical thinking and analysis would be the answer to this limitation. Almost two decades later, however, this constraint still exists.

As a solution, Watkinson (2000b) suggested that DSNs could undertake any health-related degree-level course, such as health promotion, psychology or healthcare studies, and apply the content to diabetes nursing. This can also ease the accessibility problem that exists at present relating to the available degree courses on diabetes. As noted earlier, most respondents in the present study were qualified at degree level, with 14% of them holding a degree related specifically to clinical specialist nursing practice, i.e. BA or BSc(Hons) in Specialist Practice. A considerable number of DSNs reported that studying at this level had enhanced their self-confidence and their skills and abilities to practise at an advanced level.

Almost 40% of DSNs in the present study had gained academic qualifications which, although not specifically related to diabetes nursing, had enhanced the integration of their role. These courses related mainly to teaching, counselling, management and research methods, and reflect the key components of the CNS role. These findings confirm findings by Crowley (2000) that the available educational programmes fail to prepare DSNs appropriately to correspond with the broad requirements of their multi-faceted role. These findings call for the urgent organisation of a nationally agreed course at graduate or Master's level for newly appointed DSNs.

3.5.2 Personal characteristics and skills

The Personal Characteristics and Skills Scale, developed on the basis of information derived from the literature related to the CNS role, was tested in the present study. Findings suggest that personal characteristics and role-related skills of the DSN are mutually associated with other role parameters (see *Chapter 7*). However, the literature related to the CNS role provides limited empirical evidence to support these findings. As discussed in *Chapter 2*, role theorists have contended that the level at which individuals perform their role tasks depends to a great extent on their personal characteristics and differential role skills (Brim, 1960; Biddle, 1979; Sarbin and Allen, 1968). With reference to this issue, Biddle (1979: p83) asserted that: '...the person may have difficulty in performing a role because of lack of skills or incongruence between expectations and his or her personal characteristics.'

The literature related to the role of nurses in general and that of CNSs in particular concurs with the above assertion, but empirical evidence to confirm this dynamic process is absent. However, as discussed in detail in *Chapter 7*, findings of the present study provide firm evidence that the personal characteristics and role skills of DSNs are mutually affected by their role performance. Katz and Kahn (1978: p197) proposed that '...we become what we do', and explained that an individual cannot undertake a particular role over an extended time without subsequent changes in personality. In the same way, most abilities and skills will atrophy if they are not regularly exercised.

Three underlying dimensions (factors) constitute the Personal Characteristics and Skills Scale: competence within role, organisational issues, and personal attributes. The first two items were excluded from the initial scale, as they did not load significantly on any of the factors and, thus, were not considered salient for this model. Item one related to DSNs' level of competence in the provision of diabetes care before entering the DSN post. More than two thirds (68%) felt they had an inadequate level of competence. There is general agreement that previous clinical experience in the area of specialty is necessary for the successful and quick immersion of the CNS into the role (Hamric and Taylor, 1989; Snyder, 1989; Watkinson, 1997). Many DSNs in this study reported that their previous clinical experience in the area of diabetes had assisted them to move successfully through the developmental phases. However, although clinical experience in a particular area is important, it does not necessarily denote competence in that area.

The second item excluded from this scale referred to the perceived need by DSNs to undertake further academic education related to their role. The importance of advanced education for specialist nurses is widely accepted and has been discussed in detail earlier in this chapter. More than 65% of respondents in this study perceived a need to undertake further formal education in order to maintain and/or increase their competence in the DSN role. Nevertheless, the exploratory factor analysis of data obtained from this study indicated that this item was not statistically significant in relation to this scale.

Benner (2001) contended that both clinical experience and formal education are necessary to develop expert practitioner competencies. However, results of the present study suggest that respondents did not include these within their personal characteristics and skills. Additional clarification of the findings related to the above items excluded from the initial scale was not possible in this study. For this reason, further investigation is required to test their salience in relation to personal characteristics and skills of specialist nurses. The three underlying dimensions of this scale are discussed in detail in the following part of this chapter. It should be noted that these dimensions are closely associated with each other and may often overlap.

3.5.2.1 Competence within role

The seven items loading on this factor reflected characteristics of DSNs which are associated with the degree of their competence within role. The overwhelming percentage (89%) of respondents in this study reported a high degree of competence relating to the DSN role and provision of diabetes care. The list of competencies required by CNSs in the performance of their role is enormous, considering its multifaceted nature. Worth-Butler *et al* (1994) defined competence as the acquisition of an adequate set of attributes, skills and knowledge which can be applied by individuals to do their job satisfactorily. Lillyman (1998) agrees with this definition, and adds that competence incorporates also professional judgement, reflective practice, ethics and values. The high level of competence renders the CNS able to identify areas that need improvement and to present evidence for the necessity for change. More than 85% of DSNs in the present study reported being able to defend and justify the need for change in their practice.

It is widely accepted that the advanced level of practice of CNSs requires the acquisition of critical thinking, analytical skills, clinical judgement and decision-making abilities. The first two refer to the ability of the CNS to combine practice and theory and, as Powell (1989: p825) states, to consider '...not merely the use of theory, but the concept of thinking and adding to theory while the action is occurring.' Lillyman (1998) viewed critical thinking as a composite of attitudes, knowledge and skills, while Benner (1984) added intuition to the above cognitive skills.

The two skills of clinical judgement and decision-making refer to a complex process of observing situations, of deriving meaning from the observed data, and of selecting appropriate nursing actions that can benefit patients and their families/carers, as well as other health professionals. Decision-making abilities are also required in situations where ethical issues are prominent (Hamric and Reigle, 2005). The CNS, having first-hand knowledge of patients and their families, can identify opportunities within situations involving ethical issues and resolve dilemmas.

A very high percentage (85%) of DSNs in the present study saw themselves as having a high level of decision-making abilities. Similarly, more than 80% reported that they were able to find the right solutions to different problems or situations in their practice. According to Davies and Hughes (1995), problem-solving skills of CNSs are reflected in their ability to deal effectively with complex structures of service provision of patient care. These skills are also reflected in their ability to interpret and utilise research findings, resolve conflicting situations, and initiate and implement change. The success in this process depends on the CNS understanding the care situation and having a wide theoretical knowledge base.

The incorporation of all the above competencies and skills, however, can only be achieved if CNSs have faith in their own abilities and are prepared to initiate and implement innovative ideas. These personal characteristics were identified in this study: more than 75% of DSNs reported a high degree of self-confidence and risk-taking abilities. Moreover, self-confidence was one of the main personal characteristics identified by DSNs as contributing to the achievement of implementation and integration phases, and inhibiting the occurrence of negative phases (*Chapter 5*). Patterson and Haddad (1992) perceive risk-taking abilities of CNSs as vital for their success. They add that a successful CNS is the one who is willing to take risks and face the challenges associated with breaking new ground.

Flexibility in role performance was an additional characteristic identified in this study as contributing to the enhancement of DSNs' competence within role. An overwhelming percentage (90%) reported a high degree of flexibility in their practice. The CNS is an autonomous professional responsible for coordinating and prioritising numerous commitments on a large scale, a non-traditional nurse who does not fit in the same way that a staff nurse does in a ward or unit. The staff nurse's time is planned and the day is structured around an established schedule of unit activities. The CNS, however, has to plan and manage her time according to priorities and the immediate needs of patients/carers, health professionals and institution, and should be flexible enough in role performance to be an innovator in practice.

According to Castledine (1991), CNSs, with their unique experience and knowledge of situations outside the routine nursing remit, are in an ideal position to act as agents for change and to respond appropriately to changes. The results of the present study support this assertion. However, freedom and flexibility in role performance, especially on entry into role, can result in isolation and fatigue for the CNS. Novice CNSs find it difficult to prioritise role tasks and often work long hours in order to establish an identity in the institution and prove their worth. The notion of being 'all things to all people' may be tempting for them, but hazardous to the long-term performance of their role. Therefore, the presence of a mentor is vital in helping the CNS to keep a perspective, to set priorities and realistic goals for performance, and, in this way, to make flexibility of role a positive asset.

3.5.2.2 Organisational issues

The four items of Personal Characteristics and Skills Scale loading on this factor represented respondents' ability to deal with different organisational issues and to effect change within their area of practice. The priority for the CNS as change agent is to become familiar with the structure and organisation of the work setting or institution. Equally important is to identify who has the formal and informal power to influence the system. A very high percentage (80%) of DSNs in the present study reported a high degree of familiarity with their institutions and the structure of the service provision of diabetes care.

There is a general agreement that moving change forward in a system and motivating the health staff to participate is not always easy. It is important for CNSs to acknowledge these difficulties and constraints, and accept that change cannot occur from one day to the next. This will avoid disappointment and disillusionment. Moreover, the CNSs must be able to tolerate any ambiguities or constraints deriving from the system and not allow these to interrupt the expansion of their role. However, the findings of this study do not support totally this assertion. More than 60% of DSNs reported a low level of tolerance and increased anxiety and frustration when confronted with any of the above constraints.

According to Fenton (1985), the success of CNSs depends on their ability to develop their own support system and to generate their own job satisfaction, without expecting the system to supply it. One respondent participating in Fenton's study commented that she managed to get satisfaction from:

> *'...knowing that I am able to make a difference with particular patients or staff or being able to see the change myself and not always expecting other people to come up and say something about it.'*
>
> (Fenton, 1985: p36)

Similarly in the present study, a considerable number of DSNs experienced a high degree of job satisfaction after having initiated change and improved their practice.

Motivation is another essential personal characteristic that contributes to the success of CNSs as change agents. Role theorists have highlighted the importance of motivation in the outcome of individuals' role performance. Conway (1988b) contended that highly motivated workers are able to produce high output for their organisations. More than 77% of respondents in the present study reported that their job provided them with a high degree of motivation and challenge. This was also illustrated in the comments made by respondents (*Chapter 5*), in which they described the DSN role as highly challenging and satisfying.

Negotiation skill is probably the most essential dimension of organisational issues reflecting the CNS's ability to facilitate and effect change. Change does not only occur at a slow pace, but can also be expensive, something which is not always attractive to management. Therefore, it is essential that CNSs can provide evidence for the benefits of this change and be skilled in negotiating for its implementation. More than half of the respondents in the present study rated their negotiating abilities highly. However, approximately 40% reported difficulties in negotiating with the administrative authority in favour of improvements in their practice.

This is an interesting finding, which implies that greater emphasis should be given to this area of the CNS's personal development. Negotiation skills can be incorporated into the academic educational preparation of CNSs or provided as in-service training. It should be stressed that, because change occurs across a continuum, and not at a time-limited end point, CNSs should be constantly involved in it. Moreover, as McCaffrey-Boyle (1996) maintains, effective change occurs from a group effort, and thus CNSs must be resource brokers to mobilise colleagues.

3.5.2.3 Personal attributes

The four items loading on this factor reflect the inherited attributes and qualities of CNSs that contribute to the enhancement of a competent and advanced level of practice. For a CNS, expert clinical knowledge is necessary, although not sufficient to ensure success. Specialist practice has more to do with qualities of individuals rather than their qualifications. Edlund and Hodges (1983: p503) proposed that CNSs, in order to be successful, '...must communicate their roles with statesmanship and a wide repertoire of interpersonal skills.'

Almost all (98%) of DSNs in the present study believed that they had good communication and interpersonal skills, and listened well to the concerns of others. Interpersonal competence is reflected in the CNS's ability to communicate effectively with colleagues, patients and their families in a variety of situations, from uncomplicated, routine interactions, to disagreements and conflicts. According to Hanson *et al* (2000), the key to demonstrating interpersonal skills is the CNS's ability to communicate clearly and convincingly, both verbally and in writing. The same author viewed this attribute as the second most important characteristic of a CNS, after clinical competence, in establishing collaborative relationships. CNSs who are competent in interpersonal interactions are active listeners. McCaffrey-Boyle (1996: p328) asserted that:

> *'Through eye contact and body language they* [CNSs] *portray an attitude of interest and concern. ...They are also skilled in summarising and paraphrasing elements of an interaction, resolving conflict, providing supportive counselling, and using touch.'*

Almost 93% of DSNs in the present study reported a high level of creativity relating to their role. As CNSs are expected to deal with human responses that fall outside the usual or expected range, creative and innovative skills are essential. The development of imaginative ideas and insights is essential for the continuous expansion of practice and the improvement of patient care. Finally, as noted earlier, any change or improvement occurs slowly and after a lot of effort. Therefore, perseverance and 'not giving up' are essential attributes of the CNS for success. Approximately 95% of DSNs reported that they were diligent in their efforts to bring about improvement in their area of practice. Having 'a stubborn streak that would not allow failure' was cited by CNSs in the study by Hamric and Taylor (1989) as a factor which had facilitated their role development.

3.6 Summary

The Personal Characteristics and Skills Scale developed on the basis of information derived from the literature related to the CNS role was tested in the present study. The development of this scale and the results obtained from 334 DSNs were described in this chapter. Findings suggested that the majority of DSNs rated their personal characteristics and skills highly and reported a high degree of competence within their role. Three factors were found in this scale through exploratory factor analysis: competence within role, organisational issues and personal attributes. The dimensions of this scale present a highly reliable measurement of the DSN personal characteristics, competences and skills.

The next chapter explores the second concept constituting the theoretical framework underpinning the exploration of the CNS role, i.e. work setting and organisational factors.

4

Factors influencing role development and performance

4.1 Introduction

A theoretical framework was developed from the role theory field to underpin the exploration of the CNS role. Four concepts of this framework were examined in the present study involving 334 CNSs working in diabetes in the UK: personal characteristics and skills, work setting and organisational factors, role development, and role performance. All concepts are explored in this book in separate chapters; the second concept is presented in this chapter. The review of the literature in relation to the factors that influence the role performance and development of the CNS is presented in the first part of this chapter.

The second part discusses the development of the instrument measuring the DSN work setting and organisational factors. The study findings are presented and discussed in the final part.

4.2 Review of the literature: factors influencing role development and performance

Benner's (2001) model suggests that a practitioner can perform at an expert level in a clinical situation, given innate ability and adequate educational preparation, only when he or she is 1) highly experienced; 2) motivated to perform well; and 3) has the available resources facilitating that situation. Should these conditions be different, the same nurse will perform at various levels of competence. More specifically, CNSs, whether experienced or new to the position, have unclear ideas when entering the role and several factors affect their role development and performance. These are now discussed.

4.2.1 Experience and educational preparation

The working-experience background, educational preparation, and other personal characteristics and attributes affect role performance. CNSs educated at a Master's or postgraduate diploma level but having little previous clinical experience differ from those with the same education but extensive clinical experience. CNSs in the latter group have a greater ability than CNSs in the former group in assessing situations and predicting clinical problems (Girard, 1987). Moreover, Hamric and Taylor (1989) found that CNSs' previous experience within their area of interest served as a facilitator for their successful role development and implementation. The importance of educational preparation and clinical experience to the adequate CNS role performance is explored in detail in the previous chapter.

4.2.2 Role description

The role (job) description of CNSs influences their role performance. According to Cooper and Sparacino (1990), a well-written, concise, clear and easily understood role description has the potential to increase staff and colleagues' understanding of the CNS role. A generic role description should address the basic components of the role and be consistent with the philosophy of the department of nursing regarding patients' needs, institutional goals, and nursing practice. In addition, it should be specific to a defined area of specialisation and state what services CNSs provide in that setting. However, although a generic job description is essential in providing guidance for role implementation, it should also allow CNSs to be flexible in their role performance. Priorities should be set based on the CNS attributes and the institutional and patients' immediate needs.

A clearly-documented role description which is distributed to the nursing staff, administration and others facilitates the best use of the CNS services (they know what type of assistance to seek from CNSs and when to ask for it) and justifies the cost of their services. Vague and inexplicit role description results in incongruity in role expectations imposed on the CNS from different sources within the organisation, and role conflict and ambiguity.

4.2.3 Relationships with other health professionals

Inter/intra-professional relationships also influence the role performance of the CNS. Factors such as staff resistance to change, apathy, and nurses unaccustomed to consulting other nurses have been reported as barriers to the CNS role implementation (Hamric and Taylor, 1989). In this study, one CNS reported characteristically that her greatest barrier was that experienced nurses considered themselves as specialists; not only did they not support the CNS, but they also saw her as a threat. Other factors acting as barriers have been reported, such as conflicts with physicians, team members and other health professionals.

Support has been considered as one of the basic facilitators of the CNS role. A phenomenological study, with a sample of seven CNSs working in England, aimed in part to evaluate their perceptions and experiences of their role, and factors that may influence it (Bousfield, 1997). The majority of respondents reported that lack of support from the employing organisation, nursing managers, peers, and medical staff was a major deterrent in their role performance. Moreover, most CNSs in Bousfield's study reported being clinically and theoretically better qualified than their managers. This tended to create tension and conflict between the two roles, which resulted in CNSs experiencing strong feelings of 'de-motivation'.

4.2.4 Administrative support

Administrative support is essential to the adequate role performance of the CNS, particularly for those appointed in a staff position (described later in this chapter). The CNS who has administrative support can accomplish more in a shorter period of time than the one who lacks this support. Support takes many forms, such as seeking the input of CNSs in administrative decision-making and in future plans, recognising their accomplishments, providing guidance, allowing autonomy and flexibility in role development and performance, and giving CNSs authority in the practice setting (Hamric and Taylor, 1989).

Similarly, Brown (1989) considers administrative support vital in CNS role integration and states that not only should administrators have managerial expertise, but they should also appreciate nursing care delivery issues. The role of the CNS is in jeopardy if the nursing administrator does not recognise the competence of the CNS and demonstrate confidence in and support of the role. One-third of CNSs (N = 100), participating in the study by Hamric and Taylor (1989), reported that lack of administrative support was a major barrier in the implementation of their role.

Other problems included administration limitations and misuse of the CNS role, poor leadership, and administrators doubting the worth of the role of the CNS. The study by Tarsitano *et al* (1986), aiming to compare the perceptions of CNSs and nursing administrators regarding the CNS role, showed that nursing administrators placed more importance on the research component of the role than CNSs themselves. An earlier study had reported the same results regarding the research component, but also showed that CNSs, more than nursing administrators, valued more the change-agent component (Boucher and Bruce, 1972). Such lack of congruence in role perceptions can contribute both to role strain on the part of CNSs and to disillusionment on the part of nursing administrators regarding the effectiveness of CNSs.

4.2.5 Peer support and presence of role models

The presence of peer support and role models is considered vital in the facilitation of the CNS role performance. The opportunity to share ideas, having someone with whom to compare and contrast various methods of practice, as well as collaboration in research and writing can increase the effectiveness in creating and implementing new ideas. The distinct nature of the role makes it difficult for the CNS to find someone other than another CNS to understand the problems and concerns fully and offer support, advice and practical solutions (Hamric and Taylor, 1989; Harrell and McCulloch, 1986). Having a mentor in the institutional setting, 'someone to help you learn hospital policies and the informal power source in the system' (McFadden and Miller, 1994: p31), has been cited as an essential facilitator of the CNS role performance. Support by team colleagues, clinical supervision and clinical support were some of the basic facilitators to role development identified by CNSs in the study by Newton and Waters (2001). Other supportive factors mentioned by these respondents were management support, developmental opportunities and sabbaticals, and good balance between work and home.

4.2.6 Support from the medical profession

Gaining support from medical staff is important if the role of the CNS is to survive. Traditionally, medicine has had a monopoly over other professions within the healthcare field (Humphris, 1994b). Physicians have often yearned for nurses to be their assistants and may have been upset with the autonomous route that specialist nursing has been taking. On the other hand, CNSs are not always clear about their roles and may allow the system to misuse their abilities and skills (Castledine, 1995b). They are then in danger of being called or treated as medical assistants (Bowman and Thompson, 1990). When physicians are helped to realise that the CNS role is firmly rooted in nursing and they do not wish to be seen as a new generation within the medical profession, their support will be secured. In this way, the contribution of the CNS will benefit the quality of care delivered to the patient population (Bousfield, 1997).

Kerrison (1990), in an ethnographic study of diabetes liaison nurses, explored how these nurses operated under a proxy medical model. Physicians 'promoted' the role of diabetes nurse, as it allowed the delegation of psychosocial work in which nurses claimed greater expertise. By taking on this work, nurses furthered their aspirations for professional status, while at the same time avoiding an open admission of taking over medical work. An overt confrontation with the medical staff was thus avoided. Kerrison (1990) further noted that such a confrontation would only result in the withdrawal of support by the medical profession and fragmentation of care.

4.2.7 The CNS relationships with general nurses

The type of relationship that CNSs develop with general nurses influence their role performance to either a positive or negative extent. The fact that CNSs are often in charge of evaluating patient care through clinical research and quality assurance studies sets them up as judges of the care provided. Staff nurses may then view them as a threat rather than a help, and act as an obstacle to the CNS role implementation (Bousfield, 1997).

Griffiths and Luker (1994), in a qualitative study involving sixteen community nurses, explored their attitudes towards CNSs. Although some of the respondents described CNSs as a resource, the majority saw them as a threat to their professional autonomy. This was particularly reflected in cases when CNSs were carrying out home visits or getting referrals from GPs without the approval of community nurses. Furthermore, community nurses appreciated more the role of CNSs as consultants, rather than expert practitioners. When problems arose, they preferred to draw on the CNS knowledge and bring that back to patients themselves, rather than involve CNSs in nursing care. Haste and MacDonald (1992) reported similar findings, stating that community nurses were not in favour of CNSs giving hands-on nursing care. These problems may often stem from a lack of understanding of the CNS role from the general nurses' side. Indeed, Griffiths and Luker (1994) reported that one community nurse, who had acquired some specialist knowledge in a particular area of nursing, considered the CNS to be a valuable resource, and not a threat. Therefore, as Nash (1991) agrees, a better understanding of the CNS role leaves no cause for concern and enhances cooperation between staff nurses and CNSs.

It has also been contended that CNSs can deskill other nurses if they do not apply their skills and knowledge appropriately. This may create a situation in which CNSs make all decisions regarding a specialised and complex area of patient care, keep the knowledge to themselves, and/or prevent others from taking responsibility. On the other hand, general nurses may be tempted to abdicate their responsibility and leave everything to CNSs, and subsequently not expand their knowledge and practice (Castledine *et al*, 1996; Griffiths and Luker, 1994; Marshall and Luffingham, 1998; Richmond, 2004; Wade and Moyer, 1989). This may also result in CNSs focusing on their sub-role as expert practitioners and thus neglecting other essential role components, such as educator or consultant.

4.2.8 Available time

The time available to perform all the expected activities which constitute the role of a CNS is tightly linked to the adequacy with which these activities are performed. This is remarkable, especially for novice CNSs, who often feel that they should effectively accomplish all the role components simultaneously, resulting in them being frustrated, stressed and overwhelmed. Bousfield (1997) reported that CNSs often lacked structure and direction on how to manage time and justify their role activities. Moreover, the varying expectations placed upon CNSs by the organisation, medical staff and themselves were frequently incompatible with their available time and, therefore, inhibited their role performance. Attempts to perform all the required activities at the same time often result in none of them being thoroughly and/or adequately accomplished. Therefore, it is important that realistic expectations and time-frames are agreed to assist in the accomplishment of goals and objectives.

4.2.9 Caseload size and material resources

The size and spread of the caseload or district can also influence the preferred role performance of the CNS. Newton and Waters (2001: p534) found, in a qualitative study in England, that pressure of workload was considered by 20 CNSs working in community palliative care as the largest stressor to their role development. This was described by respondents as a 'constant stream of referrals' and included factors, such as staff shortages, poor communication with other health professionals, insecurity arising from organisational changes, lack of management support and understanding of role. For example, in a large health district, travelling time reduces the effectiveness of the CNS. Wade and Moyer (1989) suggest that in such a case a greater emphasis should be given to the sub-role of educator in order to teach existing staff. In a study by McFadden and Miller (1994), CNSs considered material resources such as typing and photocopying resources, statistics consultants, audio-visual aids and library resources as valuable facilitators of their role performance. Opportunities for continuing education and services provided by professional organisations, such as position statements and standards development, were also appreciated.

4.2.10 Professional autonomy and accountability

In the study by Bousfield (1997), CNSs placed a great emphasis on the right to exercise professional autonomy, and considered it essential in the development of their role and the improvement of patient care. Autonomy refers to:

> *'...the capability of existing independently, the freedom to design a total plan of care, and the opportunity to interact on an interdependent level with other professionals. ...The enactment of authority and autonomy should perpetuate the image that nursing is an essential link in the provision of healthcare services.'*
>
> (O'Rourke, 1989: p130)

In order for CNSs to be autonomous, accountable and responsible, not only do they need to be skilful and competent, but they also need the authority to act or refuse to undertake any activities in each individual case (Parker, 1997). In Clause 4 of the *Code of Professional Practice*, the UKCC requires nurses to acknowledge any limitations in their competence and decline any duties or responsibilities unless they are able to perform them in a safe and skilled manner (United Kingdom Central Council, 1992b).

4.3 The organisational placement: staff or line position?

It has been argued that the accountability and authority of CNSs are both affected by their placement in the organisational chart (Edlund and Hodges, 1983; Holt, 1984; Storr, 1988). According to Arford and Olson (1988), organisational structure describes and dictates roles, relationships, and responsibilities by determining the formalised patterns of activities, expectations, and exchanges among individuals or groups in an organisation. Stevens (1976) pointed out the incompatibility of the multifaceted role of the CNS with the traditional bureaucratic organisational structure of healthcare institutions.

The two most common positions in the organisational structure of the nursing profession are line and staff positions. An ongoing debate exists regarding the issue of whether administrative authority should be part of the CNS's role and whether staff or line position is the most effective placement for the CNS within the organisation. Although this debate has been predominantly a North American one, it is also becoming pertinent in the UK with the establishment of Clinical Directorates, and the increasing number of CNS-manager posts (Humphris, 1994b).

4.3.1 Staff position

CNSs in a *staff position* are free of administrative tasks and have no human resource management or budget responsibility. They rely on personal and professional power derived by virtue of their clinical expertise and advanced knowledge, and also have the ability to achieve goals where others have failed to produce tangible results. The staff position allows CNSs to improve patient care directly by clinical intervention and indirectly by working in collaboration with other CNSs, members of the multidisciplinary team, and administrators, in the areas of consultation, education and research (Cooper and Sparacino, 1990; Humphris, 1994b; Scott, 1997). Moreover, by holding a staff position, CNSs are less likely to be seen as a threat by other nursing staff, because they do not have staff evaluation duties. Consequently, they are able to act as advocates for and consultants to staff members and to provide them with the needed support (Humphris, 1994b).

It has been asserted that it is not always possible for CNSs to make sufficient changes if their influence comes only through the power and authority derived from their expertise (Holt, 1984). Therefore, collaboration with and support from the administration are essential if CNSs are to function effectively in a staff position and reach the full potential of their role. Ideally, nursing administrators and CNSs should have equivalent educational preparation and should be given peer status in the organisational chart (Harrell and McCulloch, 1986; Storr, 1988).

4.3.2 Line position

CNSs who hold a staff position do not have the authority to implement their suggestions (Storr, 1988). The CNS in a *line position*, besides being an expert practitioner, educator, consultant, leader and researcher, also has administrative authority in the management of the service and its resources. The CNS combines the clinical specialist practice components of the role with the assumption of the role of head nurse, supervisor, or associate director of nursing (Cooper and Sparacino, 1990; Humphris, 1994b). Moreover, CNSs holding a line position are able to direct and motivate the nursing personnel of a unit and improve their job performance through avenues such as appraisal, sanctions, salary and promotion control (Storr, 1988). It has been reported that the line position reduces the frustrations of CNSs who do not have the legitimate power to see that their recommendations are followed (Wallace and Corey, 1983).

The primary disadvantage of the CNS being in a line position is that it is extremely difficult to balance the time spent on managerial and clinical responsibilities. Although it gives the CNS authority, all the additional management responsibilities may detract from the clinical responsibilities and draw the CNS away from the bedside. According to Holt (1984), it would be unrealistic to expect a CNS to exercise both increased clinical outcomes and excellent management at the same time. Another disadvantage of the line position is that the CNS may not have acquired graduate education in administration, and therefore will not be prepared to function in this role at an advanced level. Moreover, staff nurses may fear to expose their deficiencies in knowledge and skills to a CNS who is also their supervisor and evaluates their performance (Cooper and Sparacino, 1990; Harrell and McCulloch, 1986).

The majority of CNSs are appointed in a staff position. A study sponsored by the American Nurses Association (1986) (cited in Sparacino *et al*, 1990) showed that, of the 2327 CNSs who answered the question about their organisational position, 72% were in a staff position and 13% in a line position. However, Scott (1999) reported that of 724 CNSs, 308 (43%) were in a line position and 280 (39%) in a staff position. Although the reason for this finding was not made clear, it can be assumed that advances in the nursing specialist area and the increased competence of the CNSs result in them undertaking more administrative responsibilities as part of their role. There is no available information regarding the placement of CNSs within the organisational structure in the UK setting.

In conclusion, it is important to note that, while there have been no studies evaluating which organisational position is better, CNSs and organisations should be aware of the advantages and disadvantages in the implementation of both staff and line positions. However, Cooper and Sparacino (1990: p55) suggest that for both positions:

> *'...the key issue should be that the clinical nurse specialist's expectations and those of the organisation should fit in a position that allows for cooperation, collaboration, flexibility and congruence.'*

The ideal situation, however, would be to appoint within the same organisation some CNSs in line positions and others in staff positions.

4.4 Design and methods

4.4.1 Questionnaire design

The exploration of the role theory field showed that an individual's role performance is influenced by both contextual factors and other individuals who perform in this context. With regard to professional roles, the working environment and organisational context determine to a considerable extent the role expectations held by its members, and consequently their role performance (Biddle, 1979; Katz and Kahn, 1978).

The literature review relating to the role of the CNS revealed a number of factors associated with their performance, such as their role description, relationships with other health professionals, administrative support, available time and resources. Therefore, the purpose of this section of the study was to explore the contextual factors related to the work setting and organisational environment of the DSN. Moreover, it aimed to determine whether the DSN role performance is influenced by the above contextual or work setting factors. A quantitative approach, utilising a postal questionnaire, was adopted in this study to explore the role performance of the DSN in the UK and the factors that may influence this performance.

No relevant previously tested instrument or scale that could be adopted to examine the contextual factors related to the DSN role was identified in the literature. For this reason, this section of the questionnaire was also designed exclusively based on the information derived from the literature relevant to the topic. A six-point Likert scale format was adopted, which comprised fifteen statements (items), each expressing a different and unique dimension of the factors derived from the DSN work setting, and relevant to their role. The first five points of the Likert scale, from one (strongly disagree) to five (strongly agree), reflected the agreement or disagreement of respondents with the statements which constituted this scale. A sixth point, six (does not apply to my role), was added to this scale to identify the answers that did not fall into the five-point agree/disagree scale. For instance, this point could represent answers from DSNs who worked in the hospital setting and did not have contact with community nurses. DSNs were asked to respond to each statement by circling the appropriate number in the columns on the right.

Six of the items of this scale were negatively worded in order to avoid an agreement bias by respondents. The following statements are examples of a positively worded and a negatively worded item respectively included in this section:

Positive statement:

'The hospital medical staff are very supportive of my role as a DSN.' 1 2 3 4 5 6,

Negative statement:

'I am not satisfied with the salary I get from my job.' 1 2 3 4 5 6,

(where, 1-strongly disagree, 2-disagree, 3-uncertain, 4-agree, 5-strongly agree and 6-does not apply to my role).

4.4.2 Validity and reliability of instrument

The initial review of the questionnaire in this study was undertaken by the researcher. As a first step, a brainstorming process was adopted by including all possible items identified in the literature relevant to the purpose of each section. A rigorous review of the content of each item was then undertaken; some items which were ambiguous were reworded or omitted, and other items which measured the same dimensions were merged. An expert in linguistics assisted the researcher in this process of content clarification and reduction of items.

Subsequently, a panel of seven experts, four researchers and three DSNs working in Northern Ireland, were invited to review the questionnaire in order to establish its content validity. After the questionnaire had been critically reviewed by experts and appropriately modified by the researcher on the basis of this review, it was pre-tested in a pilot study involving 30 DSNs working in Northern Ireland. A response rate of 63.3% (nineteen DSNs) was obtained and results showed a high degree of internal consistency for the Work Setting and Organisational Factors Scale ($\alpha = 0.75$).

4.4.3 Sample

The sampling criteria for participants in this study were nurses working in Great Britain full or part time in diabetes care, with children, adults, or both, and whose title was 'Diabetes Specialist Nurse' (DSN). Access to the study sample was obtained through the *Diabetes Specialist Nurse Directory 2000* (Diabetes UK, 2000), which is the most comprehensive database available. Registration in this Directory is perceived by most DSNs to be valuable to their practice. Access to the DSN group through the above database and the sample size of this study allowed for the generalisation of findings to the overall UK population of DSNs. Questionnaires were sent to 670 DSNs working in all ten NHS Executive Regions of Great Britain. The return of the questionnaire indicated consent to participating in this study.

4.4.4 Data analysis

The 334 returned questionnaires contained valid data and were included in the analysis. The Statistical Package for Social Sciences-Version 9.0 (SPSS-V9.0) for Windows computer program was used for this purpose. For the purpose of data analysis, the negatively worded items were reversed when data were edited in the SPSS-V9.0; i.e., one (strongly disagree) was edited as five (strongly agree), two (disagree) was edited as four (agree), and vice versa. Descriptive statistics, tables and graphs were used to analyse and present the frequencies of responses. Moreover, Pearson's product-moment correlation test was used to identify any relationships between different variables. Maximum likelihood exploratory factor analysis was used to explore the underlying dimensions (factors) of the items comprising the Work Setting and Organisational Factors Scale (a detailed description of this method is presented in the previous chapter).

4.5 Results

4.5.1 Demographic details

The overall number of questionnaires returned was 341 (52.2%), of which seven were incomplete, and therefore, not usable, giving a final response rate of 51.2% (334 DSNs). Eighty-nine (26.6%) respondents were working part-time as DSNs and 245 (73.4%) full-time. With regard to work setting, 97 (29.0%) respondents were based in hospital, 43 (12.9%) in the community and 194 (58.1%) were working between hospital and community.

The majority of respondents, 53.0% (177 DSNs) were employed at H grade, 36.5% (122 DSNs) at G grade, and 8.1% (27 DSNs) at I grade. Only three DSNs (0.9%) were employed at grade E and five DSNs (1.5%) at F grade. In the UK, grading in nursing refers to the level at which each nurse practises and progresses during their career. The lowest grade for a CNS is usually at E or F, with the most senior being I grade. Grading will be soon replaced with the pay-band system under the NHS *Knowledge and Skills Framework* which is part of the new Agenda for Change initiative that is currently being implemented within the National Health Service (Department of Health, 2004).

With regard to the organisational placement, 249 (74.6%) held a staff position, that is, they had no direct responsibility in the management of service and its resources, but often provided consultation or advice regarding the organisation of diabetes care services. Somewhat less than a quarter, 74 (22.2%) respondents, held a line position (administrative authority in the management of human and/or financial resources in their own area of practice) and only 11 (3.3%) respondents reported holding a post which combined both line and staff positions. A high negative correlation was found between organisational placement and grade ($r = -.350$; $p < .001$), suggesting that DSNs holding a line position were employed at a higher grade than those holding a staff position, i.e. DSNs without managerial responsibilities had a lower grade.

With regard to the highest academic qualification earned in nursing, 44 (13.2%) respondents did not give a response. Of the remaining 290 (86.8%), 112 DSNs (38.6%) held a degree in nursing and 65 DSNs (22.4%) held a Master's degree. However, 79.0% of the 334 respondents (264 DSNs) had undertaken (or were undertaking at the time of this survey) postgraduate training related specifically to their role as DSNs. This was mainly related to National Board Courses (ENB 928 and 998). Additional information on respondents' educational preparation are presented in *Chapter 3.*

Respondents were asked whether they had a peer support group with other DSNs and, if yes, to indicate the approximate interval of time between meetings of their groups. Forty-two (12.6%) respondents did not have a peer-support group while 292 (87.4%) had, and the interval of time between the meetings of their peer-support groups is delineated in *Figure 4.1.*

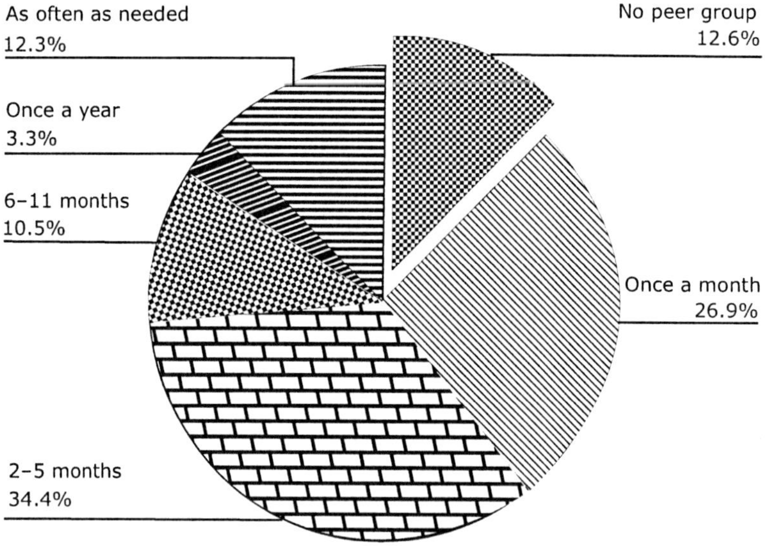

Figure 4.1 Interval of time between peer-support group meetings (N=334)

4.5.2 Work setting and organisational factors

The fifteen items combined within this section represent work setting and organisational factors related to the DSN role. These items and the statements that correspond to each of them are presented in *Table 4.1*. Items marked with an asterisk (*) accord to negatively worded statements, and their values were reversed for the purpose of data analysis and presentation. All questionnaires had no missing values and were included in the analysis.

As presented in *Table 4.2*, a wide range of responses was recorded, particularly for the last four variables (Items 12 to 15). However, the overwhelming percentage of respondents reported a high degree of support from and collaboration with other health professionals (Items 3–7 and 9). In particular, more than 93% of respondents were supported and assisted in their practice by their peer DSNs (Item 9). On the other hand, 70% of respondents reported that the size and/or spread of their caseload caused them problems in optimum performance of their role (item 10).

Responses to the sixth point of this scale 'Does not apply to my role' were obtained only for the following four items: 3 (medical staff), 4 (community nurses), 6 (hospital nurses), and 7 (general practitioners). From a crosstabulation of responses to these items with the work setting of respondents, it was found that most respondents who reported no contact with secondary care staff (hospital nurses and physicians) were based in the community. Similarly, those who reported no contact with the primary care staff (community nurses and general practitioners) were based in hospital.

Table 4.1 Items combining the Work Setting and Organisational Factors Scale and the statements that correspond to each item

Item number and code	Item statement
Job description	My job description states very clearly and precisely what my role tasks and responsibilities include
Compatibility of expectations*	I currently find that my personal role expectations/goals are incompatible with those of my employing organisation or administrative authority
Medical staff	The hospital medical staff are very supportive of my DSN role
Community nurses*	I experience difficulties in my professional co-operation with the majority of the community and/or district nurses
Healthcare team	All the members of the healthcare team within which I work are very co-operative and supportive of my role
Hospital nurses	Hospital nurses frequently ask for my assistance on different issues and problems related to their practice in diabetes care
General practitioners	Most general practitioners are co-operative and supportive of my role
Manager/supervisor*	I find that my manager (the person to whom I directly report) does not have a clear understanding of my role as a DSN
Peers/DSN colleagues	My peers/ other DSNs provide me with their support and assistance when I have problems or queries related to my practice
Caseload*	The size and/or spread of my current caseload causes me problems in time management and/or performance of my role
Professional autonomy	My role (job) provides me with professional autonomy and independence
Salary*	I am not satisfied with the salary I get from my job
Material resources	I am provided with sufficient non-clinical material resources by my organisation, such as IT support, library etc
Funding academic education*	I have difficulties in acquiring adequate funding and/or study leave to undertake further academic education related to my area of expertise
Outside professional activities	I am provided with adequate opportunities and/or funding for outside professional activities (conferences, study days, etc.)

** Negatively worded statements*

The same factor analysis procedure as that of the Personal Characteristics and Skills Scale was undertaken for the development of the Work Setting and Organisational Factors Scale. The assessment of suitability of data for factor analysis suggested that this is an appropriate method (determinant = 0.0055; KMO = 0.738; Bartlett's test of sphericity—$p < 0.001$). In addition, a large number of statistically significant inter- item correlations at the $p < 0.01$ level were reported, but none exceeded the value of $r = 0.80$.

Table 4.2 Frequency of respondents' agreement or disagreement with the items of the Work Setting and Organisational Factors Scale as rated on the six-point Likert scale (N=334)

No	Item code	1		2		3		4		5		6		Mean	SD
		Count	%	Count	%	Count	%	Count	%	Count	%	Count	%		
1	Job description	24	7.2	99	29.6	18	5.4	129	38.6	64	19.2	-	-	3.33	1.28
2	Compatibility of expectations*	45	13.5	78	23.4	24	7.2	140	41.9	47	14.1	-	-	3.20	1.31
3	Medical staff	8	2.4	28	8.4	23	6.9	112	33.5	139	41.6	24	7.2	4.25	1.12
4	Community nurses*	-	-	25	7.5	13	3.9	143	42.8	139	41.6	14	4.2	4.31	.91
5	Healthcare team	-	-	37	11.1	16	4.8	130	38.9	151	45.2	-	-	4.18	.96
6	Hospital nurses	-	-	19	5.7	5	1.5	145	43.4	138	41.3	27	8.1	4.45	.88
7	General practitioners	-	-	31	9.3	20	6.0	157	47.0	112	33.5	14	4.2	4.17	.95
8	Manager/supervisor*	59	17.7	72	21.6	28	8.4	109	32.6	66	19.8	-	-	3.15	1.42
9	Peers/DSN colleagues	-	-	16	4.8	7	2.1	125	37.4	186	55.7	-	-	4.44	.76
10	Caseload*	116	34.7	120	35.9	10	3.0	69	20.7	19	5.7	-	-	2.27	1.28
11	Professional autonomy	-	-	18	5.4	12	3.6	140	41.9	164	49.1	-	-	4.35	.79
12	Salary*	88	26.3	103	30.8	17	5.1	101	30.2	25	7.5	-	-	2.62	1.35
13	Material resources	56	16.8	111	33.2	20	6.0	100	29.9	47	14.1	-	-	2.91	1.37
14	Funding academic education*	45	13.5	82	24.6	26	7.8	135	40.4	46	13.8	-	-	3.16	1.31
15	Professional activities	38	11.4	77	23.1	20	6.0	133	39.8	66	19.8	-	-	3.34	1.33

1-strongly disagree, 2-disagree, 3-uncertain, 4-agree, 5-strongly agree, 6-does not apply to my role

* The values of these items were reversed for the purpose of data analysis. Therefore, the reversed scores are presented in this Table, i. e., 1=5, 2=4, 4=2, 5=1.

Although Kaiser's criterion suggested a four-factor solution, three factors were retained based on Cattell's scree-plot test (*Figure 4.2*), as the mean communality was 0.595. The percentage of the total variance explained by the three-factor model was 44%; the first factor contributed 20%, the second 12% and the third 12%. Factor 1 correlated at a moderate level with Factor 2 ($r = 0.219$; $p < 0.01$) and at a low level with Factor 3 ($r = 0.138$; $p < 0.01$). A moderate correlation was also found between Factor 2 and Factor 3 ($r = 0.233$; $p < 0.01$), indicating that factors constituting this scale are distinct. However, the fact that they correlate at a $p < 0.01$ level of significance indicates that they measure diverse aspects of a unique broad construct. The examination of the content of items loading on each of the three factors (*Table 4.3*) gave the following theoretical interpretation.

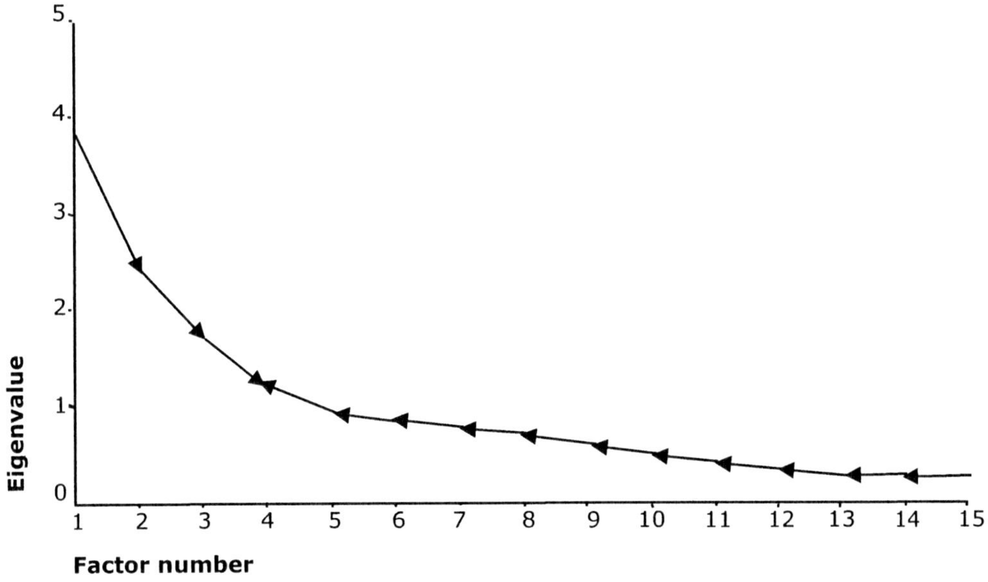

Figure 4.2 Scree plot demonstrating three statistically important factors within the Work Setting and Organisational Factors Scale

4.5.2.1 Factor 1: Collaborative working

This factor included seven items (*Table 4.3*) and described DSNs' cooperation with and support from other health professionals (see *Table 4.1* for the full description of these items). The highest loading on this factor (0.804) was reported for item 5 (healthcare team), indicating that 65% of the variance was accounted for by this factor. Item 11 (professional autonomy) also loaded highly (0.680) and accounted for 46% of the variance explained by this factor. It should be noted that the content of this item does not relate directly to collaborative working. However, these findings indicate that respondents associated their professional autonomy and independence closely with their working relationships with other health professionals. The mean value obtained from the scores of items included in this factor indicates that the overwhelming percentage of respondents were greatly supported by health professionals in their practice (Mean = 4.3; SD = 0.64). Finally, Cronbach's alpha coefficient test ($\alpha = 0.828$) suggested that the dimensions of this factor present a highly reliable measurement of the DSN collaborative working.

Table 4.3 Item loadings on each of the three factors of the Work Setting and Organisational Factors Scale

Pattern Matrix[a]

	Factor		
	1	2	3
Item 5: Healthcare team	*.804*		
Item 3: Medical staff	*.727*		
Item 11: Professional autonomy	*.680*		
Item 6: Hospital nurses	*.667*		
Item 7: General practitioners	*.603*		
Item 4: Community nurses	*.594*		
Item 9: Peers and other DSNs	*.399*		
Item 2: Compatibility of role expectations		*.838*	
Item 1: Job description		*.596*	
Item 8: Manager, supervisor		*.583*	
Item 10: Caseload		*.536*	
Item 12: Salary			
Item 15: Outside professional activities			*.912*
Item 14: Funding academic education			*.814*
Item 13: Nonclinical material resource			*.376*

Extraction Method: Maximum Likelihood

Rotation Method: Promax with Kaiser Normalisation

[a] 1-Collaborative working; 2-Role expectations; 3-Resources

4.5.2.2 Factor 2: Role expectations

The five items of this factor (*Table 4.3*) refer to the compatibility of respondents' expectations of their role with those imposed by their working environment (the description of these items is presented in *Table 4.1*). The highest loading, (0.838), as its content would also predict, was recorded for item 2 (compatibility of expectations); this accounted for

72% of the total variance explained by this factor. The dimensions of this factor present a highly reliable measurement of role expectations imposed on the DSN role ($\alpha = 0.714$).

4.5.2.3 Factor 3: Resources

Factor 3 referred to resources that facilitate role performance and the DSN's further training and continuing education and, as presented in *Table 4.3*, it included three items, the description of which is presented in *Table 4.1*. All items recorded high loadings which emphasise the importance that respondents placed on the regular updating of their knowledge and skills, as well as participation in formal academic education. Although there was a limited number of items, the dimensions of this factor present a highly reliable measurement of resources that facilitate the DSN role ($\alpha = 0.736$).

4.6 Discussion

The nursing literature relating to the CNS role provides evidence on the association of work setting factors with other role-related parameters (Bousfield, 1997; Griffiths and Luker, 1994; Hamric and Taylor, 1989; McFadden and Miller, 1994). However, a comprehensive examination of all the work setting factors influencing the DSN role identified in the literature, such as in the present study, has not been previously undertaken. The Work Setting and Organisational Factors Scale was developed on the basis of information derived from the literature related to the CNS role in general, and that of the DSN role in particular. Its test in the present study revealed that this scale presents a high internal consistency. As discussed in detail in *Chapter 7*, work setting factors were the only parameter in this study that presented a reciprocal influence with all the other parameters influencing the CNS role performance, i.e. personal characteristics and skills and role development.

The Work Setting and Organisational Factors Scale included the following three dimensions (factors): collaborative working, role expectations and resources.

4.6.1 Collaborative working

The seven items included in collaborative working described DSNs' co-operation with and support from medical and nursing staff, DSN peers and other team members, as well as the degree of autonomy and independence provided by their role. Overall, the majority of DSNs were greatly supported in the performance of their role. More specifically, an extremely high percentage of respondents (93%) in this study reported support from their peer DSNs and assistance in resolving any problems or queries related to their practice. The importance of peer support and the presence of role models in the professional growth of the CNS have been repeatedly emphasised in the nursing literature (Brykczynski, 2000; Hamric, 1983; Hamric and Taylor, 1989; Klein, 1994; McCaffrey-Boyle, 1996; Winch, 1989).

The flexible, dynamic and autonomous nature of the CNS role, as demonstrated by the present study, can however often lead to professional isolation. The disadvantage of employing CNSs cited by 49.2% of the 280 chief nurses participating in the study (McGee and Castledine, 1998) was that they could become professionally isolated. Thus, peer support helps CNSs to confront any intense emotions resulting from role stress, as well as to validate their perceptions regarding other role-related issues (Winch, 1989). It was interesting to find that the greatest single percentage of respondents in the present study, almost 30%, identified peer support and networking with other DSNs as the most helpful factor in their role development (see *Chapter 5*). This finding accords with that reported by Hamric and Taylor (1989).

In addition, as discussed in *Chapter 5*, 4.2% of DSNs in the present study cited working alone with no possibility of peer support and lack of role models as the greatest barrier in their role development. This was most notable for novice DSNs. Almost identical findings were reported by Hamric and Taylor (1989), where 5% of CNSs cited this factor as the greatest barrier. Similarly, CNSs interviewed by Bousfield (1997) stated that lack of peer support was a major deterrent to their role. Many CNSs participating in the study by McFadden and Miller (1994: p31) stressed the need for mentors in their practice and, as one commented, for '...someone to help you learn hospital policies and the informal power source in the system.'

Peer support remains crucial at any stage of the CNS role development, and, as members of a peer group, CNSs should expect to receive as well as give support. They should be committed to providing not only positive feedback, but also constructive criticism to one another. The contact among peer CNSs can be either informal, over a lunch break or through a telephone call, or can be formally arranged. The frequency of meetings may vary from weekly to bi-monthly, depending on the geographical proximity of the members of the group and their immediate needs. In the present study, the majority of respondents (34%) reported that their group met every two to five months, while for 12% these meetings were arranged as often as needed. These findings echoed those of many CNSs in the study by McFadden and Miller (1994), who expressed the need for a network of peers with whom to meet regularly for support and collaboration.

The importance of a multidisciplinary approach in the organisation of care services and effective communication among team members is widely recognised. However, differences in status deriving from historical and social factors serve as significant barriers to collaboration between professionals in a team. Other barriers identified by Castledine (1996) are related to the insecurity expressed by team members regarding the exact nature of their role and the view of themselves as representatives of their own discipline, rather than members of a collaborative team. In addition, their tendency to guard their own boundaries jealously demonstrates a lack of trust and unity. Therefore, collaboration, communication and support between the members of a healthcare team are crucial for it to function effectively and focus upon patients' needs.

In the present study, approximately 85% of DSNs reported that all members of their healthcare teams were highly cooperative and supportive of their role. Similarly, 11% reported that a supportive and encouraging healthcare team was the greatest facilitating factor to their role development. This was the second most frequently cited facilitator in this study (see *Chapter 5*). Obviously it takes time to establish trusting and collaborative relationships and the most important task for CNSs in achieving these is to make explicit the objectives and responsibilities of their role to other team members. This, in fact, applies to all health professionals working within a team. Alderton *et al* (1997: p119) investigated the impact of the DSN role in the diabetes team, and reported that DSNs played a significant part in fostering a supportive environment which helped to establish better understanding of team roles. One DSN reported, characteristically:

> *'What makes it good [effective teamwork] is learning about each other's roles. If you work with them you can learn together, which benefits the patients by sharing new ideas and challenging each other.'*

Alderton *et al* (1997) also found the DSNs' specific skills, knowledge and role activities increased team cohesiveness and improved inter-professional communication. This had allowed them to challenge medical dominance and, thus, mediate between the medical profession and others more successfully. Therefore, it can be concluded that support and recognition are not 'provided' by team members and other health professionals. Rather, they are gained by CNSs themselves through their ability to exhibit clinical and interpersonal excellence in their practice.

An extended literature has considered the patterns of working relationships between CNSs and their medical colleagues (Hamric, 1992; King, 1990; McCaffrey-Boyle, 1996; Reigle and Boyle, 2000; Spross, 1989; Watkinson, 1998). Traditionally, medicine has been considered dominant over other health professions, particularly in relation to nursing. The educational gap between nurses and physicians and their differing values about specific aspects of the healthcare continuum have often been obstacles to collaborative practice, as well as sources of interpersonal conflict. Similarly, societal expectations and gender role attributions (medicine as a male-dominated profession and nursing as female-dominated) have also contributed to the view of nurses as medics' subordinates whose role is primarily carrying out physicians' orders (King, 1990; McCaffrey-Boyle, 1996).

An additional factor in this conflict is related to the introduction of the CNS role. Physicians may perceive their authority threatened by the level of expertise that CNSs demonstrate on the basis of their advanced education and autonomous practice (Hamric, 1992). In diabetes nursing, it has become apparent that there is a blurring of boundaries between nursing and medicine. DSNs are taking on tasks that have traditionally been seen as medics' responsibility, such as insulin prescribing or ordering of laboratory tests.

The expansion of CNS practice, however, is not inevitably accompanied by conflict with the medical profession. Physicians' respect for and recognition of CNSs increase as they become aware that they are both competent and accountable, and have a complementary role in improving patient care (Reigle and Boyle, 2000). Similarly, as McCaffrey-Boyle (1996: p320) noted, '...there are many instances where CNS-physician interdependence is effective and serves as a model for others to emulate.' This was evident in the present study. More than 75% of DSNs reported a high degree of support from and cooperation with their medical colleagues in both hospital and community settings (general practitioners). Over twenty years ago when the CNS role was established in the UK, medical support was cited by CNSs participating in Castledine's (1982) study as a vital factor in the successful implementation of specialist nursing practice.

From the foregoing discussion, it can be concluded that support from and collaboration with medical staff are crucial if the CNS role is to survive. CNSs should take every opportunity to clarify their role to physicians and enable them to recognise the benefits of working collaboratively in the organisation and provision of care for patients and their families.

The CNS role performance is influenced by the patterns of the working relationship they develop with other general nurses. It has been argued that CNSs may be viewed as a threat by other nursing staff due to their expertise and involvement in the evaluation of patient care (McCaffrey-Boyle, 1996). This may, in part, stem from a vague definition of the specialist role that could result in nursing staff viewing the CNS as an intruder in their practice and, hence, being reluctant to collaborate. The majority of the sixteen community nurses interviewed by Griffiths and Luker (1994) perceived the involvement of the CNS in direct patient care as a threat to their professional autonomy. Although they appreciated the consultation role of CNSs, they preferred them not to deliver hands-on care, as they considered this to be their domain. Similar findings were reported by Haste and McDonald (1992).

An additional inhibitor to effective nursing staff-CNS collaboration highlighted in the literature is the danger of the generalist nurse becoming de-skilled (Griffiths and Luker, 1994; Marshall and Luffingham, 1998). This, as nurse managers interviewed by Wade and Moyer (1989) stated, could result in a lack of commitment on the part of other nurses who might relinquish their caring role and let the CNS take over this process. Similarly, McGee and Castledine (1998) reported that 41.7% of the 280 chief nurses in their study feared that CNSs would discourage other staff from taking responsibility. In addition, 32.8% of chief nurses regarded the issue of the CNS de-skilling other staff as a disadvantage arising from employing specialist nurses in their trusts.

In contrast, the present study revealed very encouraging results relating to the pattern of working relationships between DSNs and general nursing staff. More than 80% of DSNs reported that hospital and community nurses supported and recognised their role, and asked for assistance with different issues relating to diabetes care. However, it should be noted that these findings referred to DSNs' perceptions rather than those of their co-workers'. Thus, it is inappropriate to conclude that, since DSNs reported good working relationships with general nurses, this perception would be reciprocal. It should be noted that other studies have found discrepancies between CNSs' own role perceptions and those of community nurses (Haste and McDonald, 1992; Williams, 1993). In any case, the task of CNSs should be the clarification of their role through open communication with other health professionals if their support and cooperation is to be achieved.

An extremely high percentage (91%) of respondents in the present study reported that the DSN role provided them with professional autonomy and independence. These findings contradict those reported by Bousfield (1997), which showed that CNSs felt disempowered, and indicated that they lacked autonomy in their practice, leading to the expression of negative attitudes and feelings. They perceived the right to exercise professional autonomy and to function independently as crucial to demonstrating the benefits of their contribution to the quality of care. The capability to exist independently and the freedom to design a total plan of care are vital if CNSs are to effect change and expand their practice.

4.6.2 Role expectations

The five items constituting role expectations examined the compatibility of DSNs' expectations with those imposed on them by their working environment, that is, what DSNs expected from their role and what they actually got. In *Chapter 2* exploring role theory in relation to the CNS role, it was seen that incongruent role expectations lead to role stress and role strain, which may be detrimental to individuals' role performance (Hardy and Hardy, 1988b). Certain types of role stress (role conflict, role overload, role ambiguity) were identified in comments made by a number of DSNs in the present study when describing their role development (see *Chapter 5*). Role stress resulted from factors such as incongruent role expectations between DSNs and their institutions or managers, increased workload, and lack of understanding and recognition of their role. Many of these were included in the Work Setting and Organisational Factors Scale.

It has been asserted that a clearly-written, concise and easily understood CNS job description increases colleagues' and administrators' understanding of their role, resulting in the facilitation and support of their performance (Cooper and Sparacino, 1990). Morath (1988: p77) stressed that a job description, '...if loosely designed, can create role ambiguity, conflict, and overload, all of which will reduce effectiveness.' In the present study, 37% of DSNs cited lack of precision and clarity in their job description. The need for a commonly agreed and precise job description for CNSs was discussed in detail earlier in this chapter. This factor is highly important, due to the complex and multifaceted nature of the CNS role.

Although 56% of DSNs in this study reported compatibility between their self-expectations and goals and those of their employing organisations, a respectable 37% disagreed. In addition, almost 40% reported that their manager/supervisor did not have a clear understanding of their role and almost 18% of DSNs cited lack of support from management as the greatest barrier to their role development. Lack of understanding of their role by management was cited by 12% as the greatest barrier (see *Chapter 5*). Similar findings were reported by McFadden and Miller (1994) and Bousfield (1997). CNSs in these studies stated that, as their clinical and theoretical preparation was better than that of their managers, this tended to create tension between the two roles. Many CNSs pointed out that the CNS role '...is only as effective as nursing administration allows it to be, supports the role, and believes in it' (McFadden and Miller, 1994: p31).

Da Costa (2000) maintained that when administrators do not understand what the CNS does, they cannot appreciate the benefits of this post. Thus, the pressure to save money may outweigh any consideration of facilitating the expansion of this role. More specifically in the diabetes field, Anfield (1998) reported that the undermining and devaluing of the DSN role in her trust had resulted in a threat to remove two hospital-based DSNs and allocate their responsibilities to existing community nurses to produce savings. However, Cradock (1998: p133) noted that the blame for managers not understanding the DSN role should not be put solely upon them but '...also the whole UK diabetes nursing group.' Moreover, she criticised the current practice of DSNs and their vaguely defined role by asking:

> '...*how would you identify us* [DSNs]? *Through our agreed standards of practice? Our developing research base? Our national training programme (both preparation for the role and continuing education)? Our requirement to have a degree?*'
>
> (Cradock, 1998: p133–34)

Cradock further emphasised that if DSNs are to succeed as leaders in diabetes nursing, urgent confrontation of the above issues is required. Harrell and McCulloch (1986: p48) suggested that CNSs should meet regularly with their supervisors to set commonly agreed goals, formulate plans, and discuss progress in meeting the goals. They asserted that this strategy '...would not only lessen role ambiguity, but increase the productivity of the CNS.'

The effectiveness and job satisfaction of the CNS are greatly diminished when their scope of responsibility is too great. When they have too large a patient population to care for or when they have to cover a wide district area, Brown (1983: p161) contended that they '...feel as though they are skimming the surface of things.' Undertaking responsibilities for a large caseload may result in CNSs having less impact on care and experiencing frustration when trying to keep up with what is going on. This was supported by findings of the present study. More than 70% of DSNs reported that the size and/or spread of their caseload caused them problems in time management and performance of their role.

Salary is another issue related to DSNs' role expectations. As advanced practitioners, DSNs expect to be paid more highly for their services than general nurses. However, identifying salaries for specialist nurses within the nursing budgets is undoubtedly a major problem. In the present study, more than half (57.1%) of respondents reported being dissatisfied with the salary they were getting from their job. Miller (1995: p497) warned that:

> '...*in order to attract forward thinking dynamic practitioners, we would have to recognise these skills by high grading and monetary reward, otherwise we might lose these graduates to other professions.*'

4.6.3 Resources

The three items constituting this factor referred to resources that facilitate role performance and further training and continuing education for the DSN. Half of respondents in the present study reported that they were not provided with sufficient non-clinical material resources by their employing organisation, such as IT support, library, printing and photocopying facilities. Inadequate space or material facilities were cited by seven DSNs as the greatest obstacle to their role development. These findings are congruent with those from the study by McFadden and Miller (1994), in which CNSs considered the availability of material resources crucial to the successful implementation of their role. One commented: 'Reliable typing and photocopying are essential but rare' (McFadden and Miller, 1994: p31).

The provision of opportunities, study leave and/or funding to undertake further formal education is another vital factor impacting on the CNS role performance. Although more than half of respondents in the present study reported being provided with the above facilities, a considerable percentage (38.1%) reported they were unable to undertake further education. Moreover, funding or time constraints in undertaking further education was cited by 3% of DSNs as the greatest obstacle to their role development.

A more encouraging percentage (60.2%) of DSNs, however, reported being provided with adequate opportunities and funding for attending outside professional activities, such as conferences, study days and seminars. Four per cent identified regular updates and ongoing education as the most helpful factor to their role development. Inadequate resources to meet the needs of DSNs for increased education has been identified as a limitation to the expansion of their role (Watkinson, 1998).

4.7 Summary

The CNS role development and performance are influenced either positively or negatively by a number of factors deriving from individuals' working environment. These were discussed in this chapter and include factors such as management support, human and material resources, working relationships and communication with other health professionals and organisational placement. The Work Setting and Organisational Factors Scale, developed on the basis of information derived from the literature related to the CNS role, was tested in the present study involving 334 DSNs. Three factors were found in this scale through exploratory factor analysis: collaborative working, role expectations, and resources. The dimensions of this scale present a highly reliable measurement of the external factors influencing the DSN role.

The next chapter explores the role development of the CNS guided by a validated role development model by Hamric and Taylor (1989). Further exploration of factors influencing the CNS role is also presented.

5

Role development of the clinical nurse specialist

5.1 Introduction

The role of the clinical nurse specialist (CNS) has been described as advanced, flexible and multifaceted. Due to the complexity of the role, the CSN entering the role experiences a role development process before being able to function with maximum effectiveness. Moreover, the nature of the role and the rapid change in the health environment require a continuous change in role performance, which makes role development an ongoing and challenging process. The first part of this chapter presents a review of the literature with respect to the process of the role development of the CNS. Role development is a process of skill acquisition and change in the focus of practice through experience. Another approach to understanding the CNS role development has focused on the experiences and feelings engendered by the CNS as competence and confidence in practice are developed.

The latter approach is being explored in the second part of this chapter based on the findings of a nationwide study involving 334 DSNs working in Great Britain. This study was guided by the theoretical model by Hamric and Taylor (1989), which includes the following seven phases of role development: orientation, frustration, implementation, integration, frozen, reorganisation, and complacent. Respondents described the factors relevant to experiencing the above developmental phases. An additional phase, the transition phase, emerged from the respondents' comments. In addition, respondents identified the barriers and facilitators to their role development. Findings are presented in the second part of this chapter and discussed in the last part. Strategies are suggested for successful role implementation and elimination of negative experiences.

5.2 Review of the literature

The role of the clinical nurse specialist (CNS) has been described as advanced, complex, multifaceted and flexible in response to the needs of patients and/or institutions. It includes the following components (sub-roles): expert practice, consultation, education, research, and management (Hamric and Spross, 1989; Humphris, 1994a; McGee, 1998; Sparacino and Cooper, 1990). Newer work has focused on core competencies of clinical specialist nursing (Sparacino, 2005) which include direct clinical practice, expert coaching and guidance, consultation, research, clinical and professional leadership, collaboration, and ethical decision-making. In addition, the National Association of Clinical Nurse Specialists in the USA has further defined the CNS role as practice in three spheres of influence: the patient/client sphere, the nurse/nursing practice sphere, and the organisation/system sphere (NACNS, 2004).

The general definition of the role of the diabetes specialist nurse (DSN) conforms to that of the CNS, although it considers other significant and exclusive parameters within the diabetes-nursing speciality. According to the Royal College of Nursing (1991: p6), the DSN is '...flexible in time and location of work, permanently involved in diabetes care, innovative, and able to liaise with a variety of hospital and community personnel.'

It can be seen that the CNS, including the DSN, is a non-traditional nurse with expanded boundaries and, unlike the staff nurse or nurse manager, does not 'belong' in the same way that these nurses belong to a nursing unit. Due to the complexity of the role, the CNS entering the role or moving to a different clinical setting experiences a role development process before being able to function with maximum effectiveness. Moreover, the nature of the role and the rapid change in the health environment require a continuous change in role performance. Therefore, role development is an ongoing and challenging process for the CNS (Baker, 1979; Hamric, 1983; Hamric and Taylor, 1989). A clear understanding of this process is required not only from CNSs, but also from any individual who cooperates with them.

5.2.1 Role development as a process of skill acquisition

The role development of the CNS has been given consideration by a number of studies, particularly in the 1970s and 1980s. Holt (1984; 1987) and Baker (1987) saw the CNS role development as a process of skill acquisition and change in the focus of practice through experience.

Holt (1984) asserted that the CNS role development is influenced by individual differences in their potential and experiential background, and the uniqueness of each setting. She described seven sequential stages in which the focus of role functions evolves: 1) increasing confidence through individual direct patient care; 2) direct care and/or planning with other staff for groups of patients; 3) working with staff to change the nursing care of patients within a clinical speciality; 4) conducting and sharing small clinical research projects; 5) planning for patient care delivery changes based on experience and research activities; 6) increasing input into a higher level of healthcare delivery system; and 7) integrating all role components with increased confidence. These stages follow each other and the CNS cannot move to the next stage until competence is achieved in each of the previous stages. Moreover, these developmental activities occur over a period of years and may even encompass the whole career of the CNS.

Baker (1987), influenced by Holt's work, proposed four stages of role development based on her six-year personal experience as a CNS: 1) for the first six months, the CNS is focused on establishing baseline assessment; 2) years one and two, on establishing role identity through direct care functions; 3) years three and four, on establishing the role of change agents; and 4) years five and six, on establishing the role of consultant.

A model of clinical skill acquisition broadly discussed in nursing in the past two decades has been that of Benner (2001), which describes five levels of evolving expertise: novice, advanced beginner, competent, proficient, and expert. While Benner's work referred to registered nurses' role in general, it can be anticipated that this process is the same for CNSs as for the general population of nurses. Brykczynski (2005: pp112–113) applied this skill acquisition model to advanced practice nurses generally, noting that 'A major implication of the novice-to-expert model for advanced practice nursing is the claim that even experts can be expected to perform at lower skill levels when they enter new situations or positions.'

5.2.2 Developmental phases according to the experiences of the CNS within the role

Besides the skill acquisition process, another approach to understanding the CNS role development has focused on the experiences and feelings engendered by the CNS as competence and confidence in practice are developed. On the basis of interviews with four CNSs, Baker (1979) identified four stages of role development: orientation, frustration, implementation, and reassessment. These bear a resemblance to stages of 'reality shock' described earlier by Kramer (1974) as honeymoon, shock, recovery, and resolution. Although Kramer investigated experiences of new nursing students entering employment, her findings can also be applied to graduate nurses entering a clinical nursing speciality.

Based on her personal experience, Oda (1977) proposed three stages of specialised role development which parallel three of Baker's stages: role identification (orientation), role transition (implementation), and role confirmation (resolution). It is important to note that the role developmental models presented by Baker (1979) and Oda (1977) reflected experiences of novice CNSs who were employed for less than three years.

Hamric and Taylor (1989) undertook a study to explore the role development of CNSs with more varied experience. Their study surveyed 100 full-time practising CNSs, 42 of whom had total work experience as CNSs of nought to three years, with 58 having a total of three to sixteen years' experience. Conceptual themes from Baker's (1979) model were used to guide the exploration of CNSs with less than three years of employment. CNSs with more than three years of experience were asked, in an open-ended question, to describe their current phase of role development.

A theoretical model of seven phases of role development emerged from the study by Hamric and Taylor (1989): orientation, frustration, implementation, integration, frozen, reorganisation, and complacent. The first three phases present close similarities with the role development models proposed by Baker (1979), Oda (1977) and Kramer (1974), and correspond to CNSs with less than three years of experience, while the other four emerged from the content analysis of open-ended questions. A description of the phases constituting the model of Hamric and Taylor is presented in *Table 5.1*.

Hamric and Taylor (1989) found that the experience of these role developmental phases is not totally discrete. Rather, phases are cyclical and may recur according to prevailing situations. Moreover, there is overlap and movement back and forth depending on situations and circumstances. These findings contrast to the developmental stages in the skill-acquisition process (Baker, 1979; Oda, 1977), which were believed to always follow each other.

Table 5.1 Role development phases of the clinical nurse specialist (adapted with permission from Hamric AB, Taylor J, 1989 Role development of the CNS. In: Hamric AB, Spross JA, eds. *The Clinical Nurse Specialist in Theory and Practice*, 2nd edn. WB Saunders, Philadelphia: p48)

Role development of the clinical nurse specialist

Developmental phase	**Description and characteristics of each developmental phase**
Orientation phase	Enthusiasm, optimism, eager to prove self to setting. Anxious about ability to meet self- and institutional expectations. Expects to make change.
Frustration phase	Discouragement and questioning as a result of unrealistic expectations (either self or employer); difficult and slow-paced change; resistance encountered. Feelings of inadequacy in response to the overwhelming problems encountered; pressure to prove worth.
Implementation phase	Returning optimism and enthusiasm as positive feedback received and expectations realigned. Organisation and reorganisation of role tasks, modified in response to feedback. Implementing and balancing new sub-roles. Regaining sense of perspective. May focus on specific project(s).
Integration phase	Self-confident and assured in role. Rated self at advanced level of practice. Activities reflect wide recognition, influence in area of specialty. Continuously feels challenged; takes on new projects; expands practice. Either moderately or very satisfied with present position. Congruence between personal and organisational goals and expectations.
Frozen phase	Self-confident, assured in role. Rated self at intermediate or advanced practice level. Experiencing anger/frustration reflecting experience. Conflict between self goals and those of organisation/supervisor. Report sense of being unable to move forward due to forces outside self.
Reorganisation phase	Reported earlier experiences that represent integration. Organisation experiencing major changes. Pressure to change role in ways that are incongruent with own concept of CNS role and/or self goals.
Complacent phase	Experiences self in role as settled and comfortable. Variable job satisfaction. Questionable impact on organisation.

5.3 Design and methods

5.3.1 Questionnaire design

To examine the role development process of the DSN, the instrument developed by Hamric and Taylor (1989) was adopted for use in the present study. Permission was obtained to utilise the instrument and modify it to include all the seven developmental phases of Hamric and Taylor's model. After modifying the questionnaire, a panel of seven experts, four researchers and three DSNs, were invited to review it in order to establish its content validity. The second author participated in the panel of experts reviewing the content validity of the modified questionnaire; minor suggestions for revision were made mainly concerning grammatical errors. The revised questionnaire was then pre-tested in a pilot study with a sample of 30 DSNs working in Northern Ireland. The selection criteria of respondents in the pilot study were the same as for the main study, i.e. DSNs working full or part time in diabetes. A response rate of 63.3% (19 DSNs) was obtained. The questionnaire was revised and modified again based on the results of the pilot study (Llahana *et al*, 2001b).

Definitions of the seven developmental phases (Hamric and Taylor, 1989) were cited in the questionnaire, and respondents were asked to indicate the extent to which they experienced each phase using a five-point scale, from 'not at all' to 'to a great extent'. An open-ended question in this section asked participants to describe why they had (or had not) experienced each phase. Two further questions asked participants to indicate the approximate interval of time that each phase lasted, and whether they had experienced any of the phases more than once. However, the results of the pilot study indicated that the latter two questions should be omitted, as a high percentage of missing values (30–40%) were reported when pre-testing the questionnaire. At the end of the questionnaire, participants were asked to indicate the phase they were currently experiencing and to describe the process of their role development in case none of the indicated phases reflected their experiences. Finally, respondents were asked to list the most helpful factors and the greatest barriers in their role development.

5.3.2 Sample and data collection

The sampling criteria for participants in this study were nurses working in the UK, full- or part-time, in diabetes care with the title of 'diabetes specialist nurse'. Access to the study sample was gained through the *Diabetes Specialist Nurse Directory 2000* (Diabetes UK, 2000). Diabetes UK is a professional organisation for all health professionals involved in diabetes care and the DSN Directory is the most comprehensive database available which registers almost all the DSNs practising in the UK.

Questionnaires were sent to 670 DSNs working in all ten NHS executive regions of the UK (see *Chapter 3* for more detail). The return of the questionnaire indicated consent to participating in this study.

5.3.3 Data analysis

The Statistical Package for Social Sciences-Version 9.0 (SPSS-V9.0) for Windows was used for the analysis of quantitative data. Descriptive statistics, tables and graphs were used to analyse and present the frequency of responses. Moreover, Pearson's product-moment correlation test was used to identify any relationships among different variables. The responses to the open-ended questions were analysed by adopting a content analysis approach. This approach classifies the words in a text into a few categories according to their emerging themes and concepts, as guided by their theoretical importance (Burns and Grove, 1997; Polit *et al*, 2001).

5.4 Results

The overall number of questionnaires returned was 341 (52.2%), of which seven were incomplete, and therefore not usable, giving a final response rate of 51.2% (334 DSNs). A proportional response rate was obtained from DSNs working in all ten NHS executive regions of the UK and a breakdown of the sample of participants from each region is presented in *Chapter 3, Table 3.1*. Eighty-nine (26.6%) respondents were working part-time as DSNs and 245 (73.4%) full-time. Ninety-seven (29.0%) respondents were based in hospital, 43 (12.9%) in the community and 194 (58.1%) were working between hospital and community.

Duration of employment of respondents in their current DSN post ranged from three months to 23 years (Mean = 7.66 years; SD = 5.05) (*Figure 5.1*). For 248 (74.3%) respondents, this was the first post they had held as DSNs. The remaining 86 (25.7%) had held more than one DSN post.

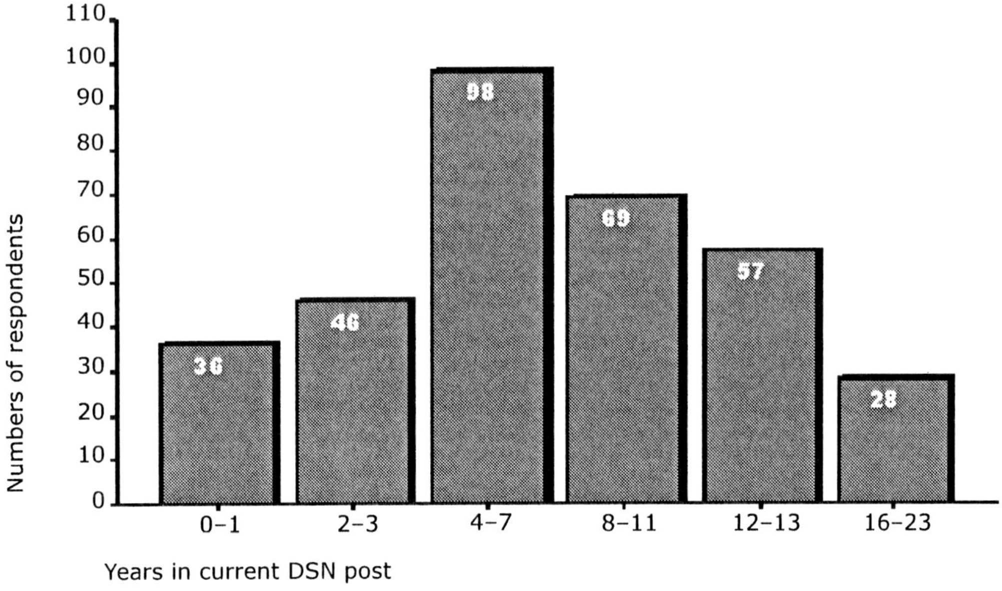

Figure 5.1 Period of time that respondents were employed as DSNs in their current post (N=334)

Most respondents, 53.0% (177 DSNs), were employed at H grade, 36.5% (122 DSNs) at G grade, and 8.1% (27 DSNs) at I grade. Only three DSNs (0.9%) were employed at grade E and five DSNs (1.5%) at grade F. With regard to academic qualifications, 264 (79.0%) of respondents had undertaken further postgraduate education related to their role, such as ENB courses; 65 (19.5%) of them held a Master's degree. A detailed description of respondents' educational preparation is presented in *Chapter 3*.

Respondents were also asked to indicate how satisfied they were with their present DSN position and, as depicted in *Figure 5.2*, the majority of DSNs (68.3%) were either satisfied or very satisfied. *Figure 5.3* presents a comparison of job satisfaction among respondents working in different NHS executive regions of the UK. Although the difference was minimal, it can be seen that DSNs working in the North West (N = 39) reported being the most satisfied with their post and the DSNs working in Scotland (N = 36) were the least satisfied.

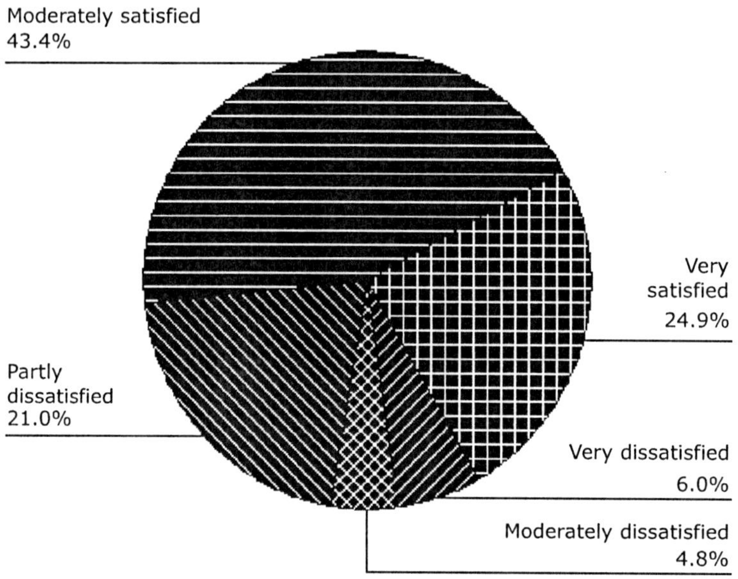

Figure 5.2 Respondents' satisfaction with their DSN position (N=334)

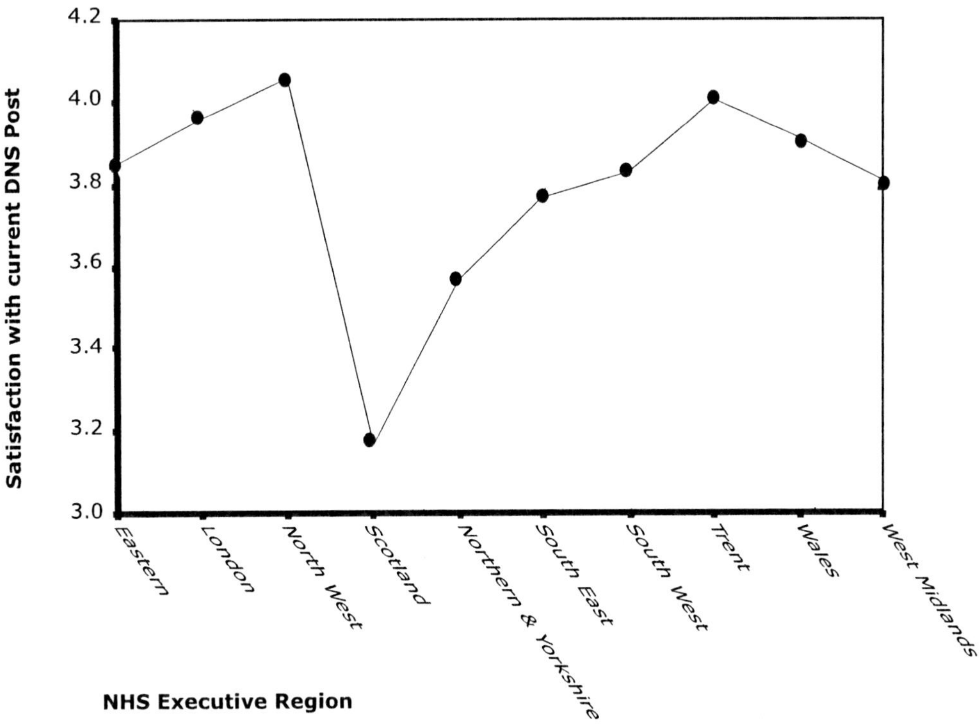

Figure 5.3 Comparison of job satisfaction among respondents working in different NHS executive regions of the UK (N=334)
[1 = very dissatisfied to 5 = very satisfied]

The results of the study indicate that the experience of role development was a highly variable and complex phenomenon. Respondents described their experiences in terms of the seven developmental phases addressed in the questionnaire, which were based on the role development model suggested by Hamric and Taylor (1989). Moreover, respondents were given the opportunity to comment on any other aspects of their role development which were not included in the above phases. By undertaking a content analysis of the comments obtained, an additional phase, the Transition Phase, emerged from the findings of this study. The definition and description of this phase are presented in the following section of this chapter.

Responses to the open-ended questions which described the reasons for experiencing (or not) each phase were divided into the following three categories:

a) Factors derived from respondents' work setting (human or material resources, support and understanding of role by management and health professionals);

b) Respondents' personal characteristics (skills, attributes and competences); and

c) Role characteristics (factors relating to the nature of the DSN role).

A wide range of responses was obtained from respondents regarding the extent of their experience of each phase as rated on a five-point scale from one (not at all) to five (to a great extent) (*Table 5.2*). With the exception of the orientation and implementation phase, no obvious differences were identified in responses between respondents working in their first DSN post and those working in their second, third or fourth DSN post. A small difference was noted in responses related to the frustration phase, indicating that the experience of this phase was stronger for respondents working in their first DSN post. Moreover, some of the reasons identified by respondents were common inhibitors or facilitators to more than one phase. Each developmental phase and reasons for experiencing (or not) each phase are described separately in the following section of this chapter.

Table 5.2 Extent of respondents' experience of each phase as rated on a five-point scale from 1 (not at all) to 5 (to a great extent) (N=334)

Developmental Phase	1		2		3		4		5		Mean	SD
	Count	%	Count	%	Count	%	Count	%	Count	%		
Orientation	18	*5.4*	66	*19.8*	71	*21.3*	120	*35.9*	59	*17.7*	*3.41*	*1.15*
Frustration	27	*8.1*	102	*30.5*	81	*24.3*	86	*25.7*	38	*11.4*	*3.02*	*1.16*
Implementation	12	*3.6*	46	*13.8*	93	*27.8*	137	*41.0*	46	*13.8*	*3.48*	*1.01*
Integration	18	*5.4*	28	*8.4*	91	*27.2*	126	*37.7*	71	*21.3*	*3.61*	*1.08*
Frozen	91	*27.2*	87	*26.0*	71	*21.3*	66	*19.8*	19	*5.7*	*2.51*	*1.24*
Reorganisation	148	*44.3*	69	*20.7*	67	*20.1*	36	*10.8*	14	*4.2*	*2.10*	*1.20*
Complacent	195	*58.4*	87	*26.0*	35	*10.5*	17	*5.1*	–	–	*1.62*	*.87*

1-not at all, 2-to a limited extent, 3-to a moderate extent, 4-to a considerable extent, 5-to a great extent

5.4.1 Orientation phase

The orientation phase presents the first developmental step in learning a new role and is characterised by enthusiasm and eagerness to prove self. A wide range of responses was obtained from respondents regarding the extent of their experience of an orientation phase as rated on a five-point scale from 1 (not at all) to 5 (to a great extent) (*Table 5.2*). More than one third of respondents (35.9%) reported experiencing this phase to a considerable extent (Mean = 3.41; SD = 1.15).

From a cross-tabulation of responses, it was found that of the eighteen (5.4%) respondents who reported no experience of orientation, nine were at present holding either a second, third or fourth DSN post. They reported being competent within the DSN role and therefore had no need for orientation and, hence, were able to move directly to the next phase. For most respondents holding their first DSN post, familiarity with setting and/or previous experience in diabetes nursing were reasons for absence or diminished strength or duration of the orientation phase.

For most respondents who held either a second, third or fourth post and had experienced this phase, the knowledge and familiarity with the role helped them to move through it very quickly. The majority stated that their orientation was not related to the role itself but rather to the new practice setting, institution, healthcare team, and/or patients. As described later in this chapter, these respondents had in fact experienced a transition phase which, although similar to the orientation phase, presents distinct characteristics.

Almost half of respondents in this study related their experience of an orientation phase to the newness of the DSN post in their institutions and the need to establish, promote and prove the importance and benefit of the role. This is illustrated in the following comment:

> *'Twenty years ago, a DSN was rare. We were pioneers and it was an exciting new role that no one had done in this area. We had to prove this role was of worth, and that it was needed and what was needed.'*

Approximately one third of respondents who reported positive experiences of this phase reported that an induction programme into the role and work setting had been arranged by DSN colleagues and/or managers. Furthermore, as illustrated in the following comments, support and recognition of role were significant factors in the occurrence of this phase:

> *'I joined a happy, established and experienced team who were willing to listen to new ideas and support new staff.'*

> *'I worked with an extremely enthusiastic and innovative consultant diabetologist... He strongly supported the idea that a diabetes service could not be run sufficiently without a specially trained nurse'.*

With respect to personal characteristics, most respondents reported that, by undertaking a new post, they felt energetic, enthusiastic and interested in developing and advancing their role. They also felt keen and eager to effect change and 'make a difference' in the care of people with diabetes.

On the other hand, lack of mentors was cited as a factor that slowed down the progress of many respondents' role development, with one DSN commenting characteristically, '...I did not know what I did not know'. Moreover, lack of support, professional jealousy, as well as lack of understanding of the DSN role, were reported as inhibitors to moving quickly through the orientation phase. One DSN commented:

> *'This was a new post in the health authority. I had no direction or role model to follow. I set up the post from nothing and had the feeling of being a threat to medics especially because they had doubts about role.'*

5.4.2 Frustration phase

Feelings of depression, discouragement and inadequacy accompany the occurrence of this phase. A wide range of responses was obtained regarding respondents' experience of the frustration phase (*Table 5.2*). The majority (30.5%) reported a limited experience of this phase (Mean = 3.02; SD = 1.16).

Factors deriving from respondents' work setting were major determinants of absence or limited experience of this phase. They included support from and good working relationships with peers, team members, and other health professionals, as well as working in a positive environment. Support and recognition of role by management were cited by many respondents, with one stating, 'I have a good manager who allows discussion of feelings so that a problem does not develop and she is always encouraging'. In particular, one of them noted that '...having a manager who has been a DSN helps'.

Personal characteristics, such as determination, strength of character, enthusiasm, optimism, tolerance, good planning abilities, setting realistic expectations for role performance and recognising self-limitations contributed to the elimination of frustration for many respondents. Expertise obtained from previous DSN posts was also cited, while one respondent related the absence of frustration to the DSN role which was '...always varied, interesting and rewarding'.

In contrast, most respondents who experienced a frustration phase related this to the lack of support, understanding and recognition of the value of their role. This is illustrated in the following comment:

> *'When I was overwhelmed by sheer numbers, covering a large rural area and towns, and both children and adults, my prepared statement on increased population figures and increase in diabetes was "lost" by management. I was considered inefficient.'*

Further factors that caused the frustration phase were related to the absence of role models and isolation of respondents as they worked alone due to inadequate DSN staffing. Similarly, ten respondents reported lack of peer support and conflict with other DSN colleagues, with one stating:

> *'The DSN supervising me was obviously threatened by my academic qualifications and capability once the induction phase was completed. I was not included in research and was given no opportunity to expand my knowledge base. I was made to feel incapable, inferior, and made to appear less knowledgeable in every possible situation.'*

Incongruence of role expectations and conflict between respondents and other parties or the employing organisation also contributed to the sense of frustration. 'I was expected to be excellent in my job immediately' noted one respondent, while another felt pressured as '...patients want things done immediately'.

The second most frequently mentioned reason that caused frustration was related to time limitations due to increased workload. Having a part-time DSN post also caused time constraints and frustration, because, as one respondent noted, 'I am contracted for 23 hours while the workload far exceeds this.' Staff shortages, inadequate facilities (limited space, clerical and IT support) and unavailability of funding for further training and education were cited by almost one third of respondents. Some respondents reported that two or more of the reasons above contributed to the experience of this phase. This was most notable for those who reported a great deal of frustration, as in the following example:

> *'Poor management! When I arrived I did not have a desk or a phone in any office and was trying to sort this out, together with orientation to the hospital and the area* [this respondent held a second DSN post]. *I was immediately being given referrals, 25 in the first month mostly urgent, as there had been a gap from the previous DSN retiring. After the bad start, workload pressures continued to the present day and are still increasing.'*

Finally, five respondents saw this phase as natural, occurring on 'bad days', and as something that 'comes and goes' occasionally, depending on prevailing circumstances. A number of respondents reported on how they managed to move forward from the frustration phase. This had happened either by chance (for example the resignation of a non-supportive colleague or manager) or had been instigated by respondents themselves. Self-education and undertaking study days to increase their knowledge base were reported strategies. Similar strategies included moving to another DSN post or undertaking professional development, as reflected in the following comment: '...I went to do some research part-time which I found to be a very useful learning curve.' However, one respondent used the coping strategy of acceptance to overcome the frustration phase:

> *'Heavy workload made me cope only and not get satisfaction from my job. I accepted that there was no chance of making changes or others becoming interested in problems.'*

5.4.3 Implementation phase

Optimism, enthusiasm and feelings of being accepted occur with this phase. As presented in *Table 5.2*, only twelve (3.6%), six of whom held a second DSN post and one who held a fourth DSN post, reported no experience of the implementation phase. Three of them reported that, due to their previous expertise in role, they felt very confident and were very well accepted into their new team. Of the remaining four DSNs in this group, three were just entering this phase (they had been employed for three months), while one reported being still in the frustration phase and saw no change in the new post: '...role still repetitive and I am not being involved much in local issues.'

Absence or limited experience of this phase was often attributed to the short time in post or the extended duration of orientation and frustration phases. However, factors deriving from respondents' work setting were the main obstacles to the occurrence of the implementation phase. These were lack of support, acceptance and understanding of role by management and other health professionals. 'I was left on my own to cope' said one DSN, while another found it '...difficult to implement new ideas as the consultant was strict in old fashioned ways.'

Time pressures due to increased workload and restrictions on resources (human and material) were further reasons which inhibited the occurrence of implementation. 'Too busy to move on trying to deal with the everyday overwhelming caseload...' felt one respondent.

On the other hand, for more than half of respondents, experience of this phase was attributed to the initiation and successful implementation of a project or initiative. One respondent reported '...choosing projects which can be implemented in a short time span and evaluating results fairly quickly' as a strategy to reach the implementation phase. The strength of this phase arose from the support, recognition and positive feedback from peer DSNs, management, health staff and patients, as well as good communication and coordination. This phase was even stronger when the manager was a specialist nurse, as for the following respondent: 'The employment of the DSN team manager encouraged expansion of our role and raised the profile of our team within the trust.' Setting realistic goals and '...realisation by all members of the team that we needed to be focused' were also cited. In addition, continuous audit and evaluation of practice setting, role and self contributed significantly to this phase. Two respondents reported:

> *'Each year we specify in the annual report what plans we want to implement for the following year. It is rewarding to review outcomes at the end of the year';*
>
> *'I re-evaluate my role and use reflective practice to identify areas for change. Clinical supervision is an essential part of my practice.'*

Other reasons identified by respondents as contributing to the implementation phase were learning and gaining expertise and confidence from experience and attendance at academic courses and study days. A smaller percentage of respondents felt that their increased self-confidence and better decision-making abilities due to advanced knowledge, as well as optimism, enthusiasm, motivation, perseverance, and a 'sense of perspective' related to the role, helped them to reach implementation.

5.4.4 Integration phase

Self-confidence, assurance and continuous challenge characterise this phase. The results obtained relating to the extent of experience of this phase were similar to those of the implementation phase, with a wide variety of responses (*Table 5.2*). Forty-six (13.8%) respondents reported absence or a limited experience of an integration phase. The main reason for absence or a limited experience was related to the short period of employment in a DSN post, as the majority of respondents had been employed for less than three years.

Other reasons were related to time limitations resulting from staff shortages, increased workload or part-time employment, constraints on resources, as well as lack of support, co-operation and negative attitudes of other health professionals. Respondents reported that, although they had acquired an advanced level of practice, these constraints did not allow them to become innovative and effect change. One DSN commented:

> *'My role is well-recognised and respected by peers for the service I provide and is appreciated by patients, but limited resources impede undertaking new projects and expansion of practice.'*

Staff shortages and/or inadequate DSN coverage were also mentioned, with one respondent stating, '...not enough staff over many months have left remaining DSNs working at crisis levels.' Not only did the above limitations impede expansion of practice, but they also resulted in respondents' dissatisfaction with role, with one noting, 'I am rapidly losing interest in my job and role.' Four respondents reported two or more reasons which acted simultaneously against integration, as in the following example:

> *'I have no opportunity to develop as there is lack of time allowed for study leave, lack of resources, insufficient staff, and lack of backup by management to provide me with support to develop position and role.'*

On the other hand, reasons relating to the occurrence of this phase were similar to those identified in implementation. However, respondents reported a higher level of practice, self-confidence, and competence in the integration phase. The majority of respondents felt they had reached this phase after the successful implementation of a major project and 'seeing ideas in action' which had brought improvement in the area of their practice. This included projects such as development of nurse-led clinics and expansion of primary care services, setting up and delivering diabetes teaching programmes and prescribing protocols. Respondents had received positive feedback, their opinion was respected and they were able to influence decisions regarding the organisation and provision of diabetes care. The recognition of their expertise was reflected in the high frequency with which other health professionals and management sought their advice and consultation on different issues related to diabetes. One DSN stated:

> *'Positive feedback generally indicates patient and colleague satisfaction. I am frequently asked for advice. I have been also asked to contribute to policy-making across the trust.'*

Promotion and undertaking positions with higher responsibility were also mentioned. Reaching this phase was also attributed to expertise gained through clinical experience, ongoing education and 'keeping up to date with current trends', as well as continuous evaluation of self-competence within role. One respondent commented:

> *'After six years in post, I feel that I practise at an advanced level. I continuously review and reflect upon my practice and evaluate provision of care to implement innovations.'*

Twenty respondents assigned the experience of this phase to their self-confidence, optimism, motivation, role competency, interpersonal skills and 'perseverance in achieving planned goals and personal expectations'. A number of respondents related integration to the multifaceted, challenging and satisfying nature of their role. Characteristics such as autonomy, independence, flexibility and 'freedom from usual barriers for development' were cited. 'I felt this job totally fulfilling, which enabled me to use all my qualifications and special skills,' commented one respondent. However, as illustrated in the following comment, autonomy itself was not always effective in the expansion of role:

> *'As an autonomous practitioner it can be beneficial as well as frustrating in my role. I can initiate projects, but resources and support from other professionals do not always follow.'*

Finally, a number of respondents reported 'movement in and out' of this phase as roles evolved throughout years, mixed with feelings of frustration or complacency at times. One respondent noted that '...There are occasional knock-backs, but generally practice grows and expands—some problems are releasing tasks to take on new roles.'

5.4.5 Frozen phase

This phase occurs in the presence of incongruent role expectations. A wide variety of responses were obtained by respondents regarding their experience of a frozen phase (*Table 5.2*). Most respondents (53.0%) reported either absence or a limited to moderate extent of this phase (Mean = 2.51; SD = 1.24).

The main reason relating to the absence of this phase was the short period of time respondents were employed in their present post and who, thus, had not reached an advanced level of practice. Recognition, support and encouragement, particularly from nursing management, and working within a supportive and well-organised team were the main reasons related to its absence. Compatibility of role expectations between respondents and their employing organisations/managers was also mentioned. Other reasons were related to respondents' personal characteristics such as enthusiasm, perseverance, determination, problem-solving abilities, competence and confidence within role. One DSN stated: 'It is very rare that I feel like this. However, if there is opposition to a new project I would have the ability to present evidence and support my case.' Fifteen respondents reported that they were able to overcome constraints and move practice forward by working within a supportive and well-organised diabetes team. Another respondent cited autonomy and '...encouragement to develop my role the way I wanted' as an inhibitor of this phase.

Respondents who had experienced a frozen phase reported feeling confident and competent within their role, and practising at an advanced level. However, different obstacles deriving from their work setting made them feel 'stuck' and 'unable to move forward'. These obstacles were similar to those identified in the frustration phase. A high correlation ($r = 0.470$; $p < 0.001$) was found between frustration and frozen, confirming the similarity of factors causing these phases. Most respondents attributed this phase to the lack of support, recognition and understanding of their role by management and health staff, the incongruence of role expectations, as well as the view of diabetes care 'at a low profile on management agenda'. The following is a typical comment made by this group of respondents:

> *'Although very experienced and therefore confident in my role, I feel that the management let me get on with it and there are times when showing some interest would be appreciated.'*

Increased workload and constraints on resources were mentioned by almost 30% of respondents, with one stating, 'I have researched the need, identified action plans, but do not have resources to implement.' Other reasons included absence of career prospects, mostly notable for respondents working part-time, as they '...are not always given the senior grades or opportunities for further education, research, conferences etc, that full-time staff are given'.

Finally, as in frustration, a limited number of respondents who reported a great extent of experience of frozen phase identified more than one reason acting simultaneously. This is illustrated in this comment:

> *'Conflict within the team is causing problems. Workload is too high and totally revolves around patients. There is no real scope for individual creativity, development or research. Very frustrating!* ...[There is] *very little support, no clinical supervision, DSN meetings but no peer support. I am about to leave my present position as a result of the above.'*

5.4.6 Reorganisation phase

Feelings of stress and anxiety accompany the occurrence of this phase due to pressure to conform to organisational requirements. Almost 45% of respondents in this study reported absence of a reorganisation phase (*Table 5.2*). As in the integration and the frozen phases, most respondents who were employed in their posts for less than three years had not experienced this phase. In addition, a considerable percentage of respondents reported that there had been no changes in the organisational structure of their institutions. For other respondents, these changes had not affected their role, as the scope of change was compatible with their expectations. One DSN reported: 'Fortunately, I have had very little experience of this phase. DSNs in my institutions are usually looked to to instigate change rather than have change forced on us.'

Other reasons for absence or limited experience of this phase were attributed to the support and autonomy for role performance provided by administration. Moreover, ten respondents stated that their good working relationships and the discussion of different issues with colleagues had not allowed any organisational changes to have a negative impact on their role. 'Most projects are discussed as a team where every member participates, and then protocols are put in progress,' commented one respondent. Confidence and competence within role, as well as ability to 'argue point' and negotiate with administration, had also inhibited the occurrence of this phase. One DSN noted:

> *'I have always been able to engage managers and other health professionals regarding any changes needed in my role. Therefore, any pressure from them is minimal and compatible to my expectations.'*

For respondents who had experienced this phase, reorganisation had created changes to which they had to adjust and adapt. Pressure was exerted on respondents to assume new responsibilities within their role (or exclude others), not congruent with their expectations, such as undertaking a great amount of managerial activities. Finally, frequent reorganisation of diabetes care services and changes in management structure were reported by eleven respondents as contributing to this phase. This had caused confusion relating to role responsibilities and poor communication between different health professionals and/or departments. One respondent stated characteristically:

> *'The trust has merged, un-merged and changed name and service provision twice in a space of two years. I spent lots of time having to adapt to this change and had no opportunity to develop my role during this period.'*

5.4.7 Complacent phase

In this phase the challenge to effect change is absent. None of the respondents in this study reported having experienced a complacent phase to a great extent, while more than half (58.4%) reported absence of it (*Table 5.2*). Short time in employment was one of the reasons for absence of this phase. However, the majority of respondents attributed its absence to the nature of diabetes nursing, which is 'too innovative and challenging to bring complacency'. 'Each patient represents a new challenge,' noted one DSN, while another reported: 'Diabetes care and research is changing so much that there is never a feeling of stagnation.' Respondents had 'a lot to learn' through a continuous update of knowledge and skills, as well as constant reappraisal of their role.

Regarding personal characteristics, respondents perceived their motivation, competence, enthusiasm, innovation and constant search for new ideas and challenges as inhibitors to the complacent phase. Many respondents reported that their self-pride would not allow them to become complacent. 'It would be very easy to settle in this phase but I am determined not to!' stated one DSN. Moreover, the desire to provide a quality service for patients, their families and other health professionals helped respondents to maintain a broad focus of performance. The strategy chosen by ten respondents to avoid feelings of complacency was attendance at academic courses and study days. One DSN stated: 'You do become comfortable in a role, but you also need to challenge yourself. I am now undertaking an MSc to improve my practice and provide me with a challenge.' The elimination of this phase was also attributed to the multifaceted, challenging, satisfying and rewarding nature of the DSN role which '...always provides a broad spectrum of new things to do'. Respondents perceived this as '...an exciting role with constant changes and opportunities', which '...inspires one to look further and consider varying aspects of care'.

Only 15% of respondents had experienced a complacent phase either to a moderate or to a considerable extent. One reason for this was related to the length of time within role, which made DSNs feel 'comfortable' and 'sit back for a while'. Moreover, this phase occurred when change of post was considered, as for this DSN: 'I am looking for a new job. This has impacted on my desire to search out new challenges in my current role.' Furthermore, personal or family commitments had contributed to this phase: 'I experienced a complacent phase between children when motherhood was more important than career.' Other reasons were lack of support, increased workload and constraints on resources, which inhibited change and challenge. Respondents had adopted a 'why bother' attitude for the period of time that these constraints lasted, as they could not see 'a way through' them.

However, short intervals of a complacent phase were perceived by a considerable number of respondents as a pleasant phase to be in from time to time. They had experienced short intervals of this phase and had seen this as a 'recharging' and 'stand still and reflect' period of time. This was most notable for respondents who had implemented a stressful project successfully and, therefore, saw this phase as 'consolidation' and '...allowing myself time to enjoy achievement'. One DSN commented:

> *'Eventually, the department has reached a time of stability regarding staffing numbers and workload. I have no desire to undertake more responsibilities and goals. I enjoy the time being able to cope for a change.'*

Finally, five respondents felt it would be nice to experience 'short spells' of complacency, as their job was often 'overwhelming'. 'Wish we had time "to come up for air"!' stated one of them.

5.4.8 Transition phase

Respondents in this study were asked to indicate any other aspects or experiences of their role development which were not included in the seven phases addressed in the questionnaire. An eighth phase, the transition phase, emerged from the analysis of respondents' comments. Characteristics of this phase were also present in the comments of respondents relating to the orientation phase. Transition was a typical phase for experienced DSNs who held either a second, third or fourth DSN post (n = 86) to report experiencing.

The definition and basic characteristics of the transition phase are as follows. Transition is characterised by enthusiasm, excitement and eagerness in bringing about improvement in the area of practice when beginning a new DSN post. The DSN reports self-confidence, assurance, competence and advanced level of practice within the role. Previous experience and expertise are recognised by team members and other health professionals in the new setting. Feelings of anxiety are related to orientation into a new work setting rather than to the DSN's knowledge base.

This phase presents similarities to the orientation phase suggested by Hamric and Taylor (1989). However, individuals who experienced a transition phase reported confidence and competence within role, advanced level of practice, as well as previous experiences of implementation and/or integration phases. 'This was my second post as a DSN, therefore, I entered this post with more confidence and enthusiasm,' noted one respondent.

Respondents experiencing the transition phase reported feeling anxious when undertaking a new post due to the change of setting rather than their knowledge base. That is, they were concerned about becoming familiar with the organisational structure and administration, and establishing working relationships with team members, other health professionals, and patients and their families. The duration of this phase ranged from a few days to six months, as illustrated by the following respondent who held a second DSN post: 'It was at least six months after my appointment before I had built up a thorough knowledge of local working practice, support systems and geographical layout.'

For most respondents the change to another DSN post was their own choice. Therefore, they felt enthusiastic, excited and keen to make changes that would bring improvements in the provision of diabetes care in the new setting. Their expertise allowed them to evaluate and assess areas that needed change, as well as to suggest appropriate strategies and initiate implementation of change. 'I was able to see clearly changes that needed to be made,' reported one DSN. Similarly, two other respondents commented:

> *'I was very excited to be the first DSN in my area. Being an experienced DSN, I was able to make many changes and implement many ideas very quickly',*
>
> '[I was] *bringing eight years of experience to a new post.* [I was] *excited for being able to mould the job as I see it.'*

A smaller number of respondents reported that they had been appointed to their new DSN post with the aim of undertaking a new project. 'I was brought into this job to make changes and have had support in doing so' noted one respondent. Two others had been employed at the time of the opening of a diabetes centre and, therefore, had the opportunity to use '...immediately all the expertise gained in the previous post'.

The transition phase was also reported by a small number of experienced DSNs who had moved to another work setting within the same post, for instance from secondary to primary care. They perceived more prospects for role development in the new setting and felt being '...able to use all [of their] qualifications and special skills'. Characteristically, one respondent stated:

> *'I worked alone in the community at first. Since 1990, I have moved into the hospital.* [I found] *more scope for change here, although I was anxious at first about commitment to the wards.'*

Respondents' previous experience and expertise helped them to gain recognition and become an integrated part of the new team shortly after their employment. They were able to establish good working relationships and communication within their new setting and 'put their ideas into action'. The majority of the 86 respondents who had held more than one DSN post described experiences matching the transition phase.

5.4.9 Correlation between developmental phases

The relationship between the seven developmental phases of the model devised by Hamric and Taylor (1989) and tested in this study was investigated using Pearson's product-moment correlation test (*Table 5.3*). On the basis of the results obtained from this correlation matrix and the definition of each phase, the developmental phases were categorised in two distinct and non-correlated groups as positive phases (implementation and integration) and negative phases (frustration, frozen, reorganisation and complacent). The exception was the orientation phase, which was not included in any of the categories and did not correlate with any other phase. This, as described earlier in this chapter, can also be confirmed from the comments received by respondents related to this phase. Some DSNs associated the orientation phase with positive feelings and experiences, and others with negative.

Significant correlations were seen among the negative developmental phases, with the frustration phase being positively correlated with the other three negative phases. The strongest association was between frustration and the frozen phase. These findings indicate that DSNs who experienced the early negative frustration phase were more likely to experience subsequent negative developmental phases. The complacent phase also correlated at the $p < 0.001$ level of significance with the frustration, frozen and reorganisation phases. Conversely, integration showed a weak, but statistically significant, negative correlation with frustration, indicating that the stronger the experience of frustration, the weaker was the experience of integration. Integration was also positively correlated with implementation.

Table 5.3 Examination of relationships between developmental phases using Pearson's product-moment correlation test (N = 334)

Orientation Phase	Pearson r Sig.	*1.000*						
	p	.						
Frustration Phase	Pearson r Sig.	*.080*	*1.000*					
	p	*.143*	.					
Implementation Phase	Pearson r Sig.	*.060*	*-.048*	*1.000*				
	p	*.272*	*.378*	.				
Integration Phase	Pearson r Sig.	*.000*	*-.110**	*.326****	*1.000*			
	p	*.998*	*.045*	*.000*	.			
Frozen Phase	Pearson r Sig.	*.022*	*.470****	*-.047*	*.103*	*1.000*		
	p	*.695*	*.000*	*.395*	*.060*	.		
Reorganisation Phase	Pearson r Sig.	*-.084*	*.312****	*.040*	*.095*	*.351****	*1.000*	
	p	*.127*	*.000*	*.463*	*.104*	*.000*	.	
Complacent Phase	Pearson r Sig.	*.040*	*.240****	*-.034*	*.122* .026*	*.295****	*.292****	*1.000*
	p	*.465*	*.000*	*.531*		*.000*	*.000*	.
Developmental Phase		Orien/on Phase	Frustr/on Phase	Imple/on Phase	Integr/on Phase	Frozen Phase	Reorg/on Phase	Comp/nt Phase

* Correlation is significant at the 0.05 level (2-tailed)

*** Correlation is significant at the 0.001 level (2-tailed)

5.4.10 Order of experience of developmental phases

One of the objectives of the study by Hamric and Taylor (1989) was to determine the duration and order of occurrence of the developmental phases. No particular sequence of their occurrence was found, and many CNSs noted an overlap between and recurrence of these phases.

The duration of time that each phase lasted could not be determined in the present study as respondents found it hard to specify. Most respondents in the pilot study did not answer this question. An alternative approach in the main study was to ask respondents to rank the order in which they had experienced these phases. For the purpose of data editing and analysis, the phases were coded as follows: 1-Orientation, 2-Frustration, 3-Implementation, 4-Integration, 5-Frozen, 6-Reorganisation, 7-Complacent.

Results are presented in *Table 5.4* and illustrated in *Figure 5.4.* As seen in *Table 5.4*, the means of the order of developmental phases, based on the above coding, indicate that these phases occurred in sequence for the majority of respondents. An exception was the frustration phase, which occurred third (Mean = 3.77; SD = 2.48), while the implementation phase occurred second (Mean = 2.64; SD = 1.34). Orientation always occurred first for all DSNs who experienced this phase (94.6%). A considerable number of respondents, as indicated by the eight section in *Figure 6.6*, indicated that they had experienced most phases more than once, with the exception of orientation and implementation.

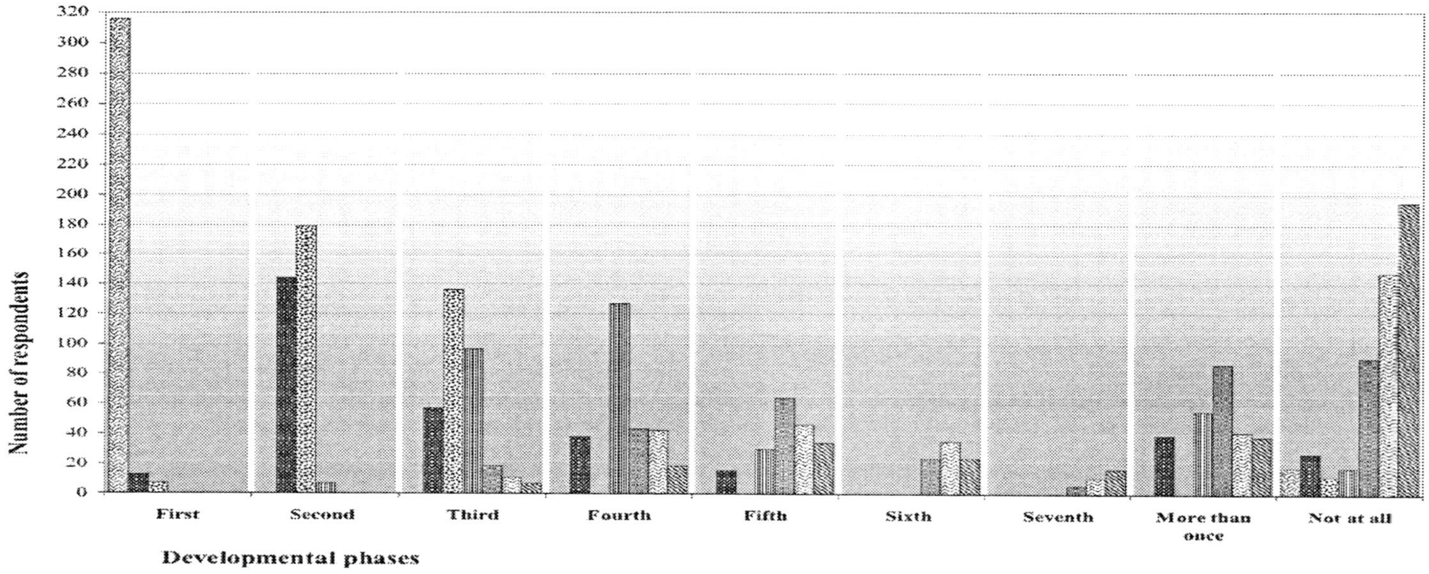

Figure 5.4 Order of experience of developmental phases (N = 334)

Table 5.4 Order of experience of the developmental phases (N=334)

Order of experience of each phase	First		Second		Third		Fourth		Fifth		Sixth		Seventh		More than once		Not at all		Mean	SD
	n	%	n	%	n	%	n	%	n	%	n	%	n	%	n	%	n	%		
Orientation	316	94.6	-	-	-	-	-	-	-	-	-	-	-	-	-	-	18	5.4	1.43	1.81
Frustration	13	3.9	144	43.1	57	17.1	38	11.4	16	4.8	-	-	-	-	39	11.7	27	8.1	3.77	2.48
Implementation	7	2.1	179	53.6	136	40.7	-	-	-	-	-	-	-	-	-	-	12	3.6	2.64	1.34
Integration	-	-	7	2.1	97	29.0	127	38.0	30	9.0	-	-	-	-	55	16.5	18	5.4	4.69	1.99
Frozen	-	-	-	-	19	5.7	43	12.9	64	19.2	24	7.2	6	1.8	87	26.0	91	27.2	6.74	2.05
Reorganisation	-	-	-	-	11	3.3	42	12.6	46	13.8	35	10.5	11	3.3	41	12.3	148	44.3	7.12	2.05
Complacent	-	-	-	-	7	2.1	19	5.7	34	10.2	24	7.2	17	5.1	38	11.4	195	58.4	7.75	1.79

1-Orientation phase, 2-Frustration phase, 3-Implementation phase, 4-Integration phase, 5-Frozen phase, 6-Reorganisation phase, 7-Complacent phase

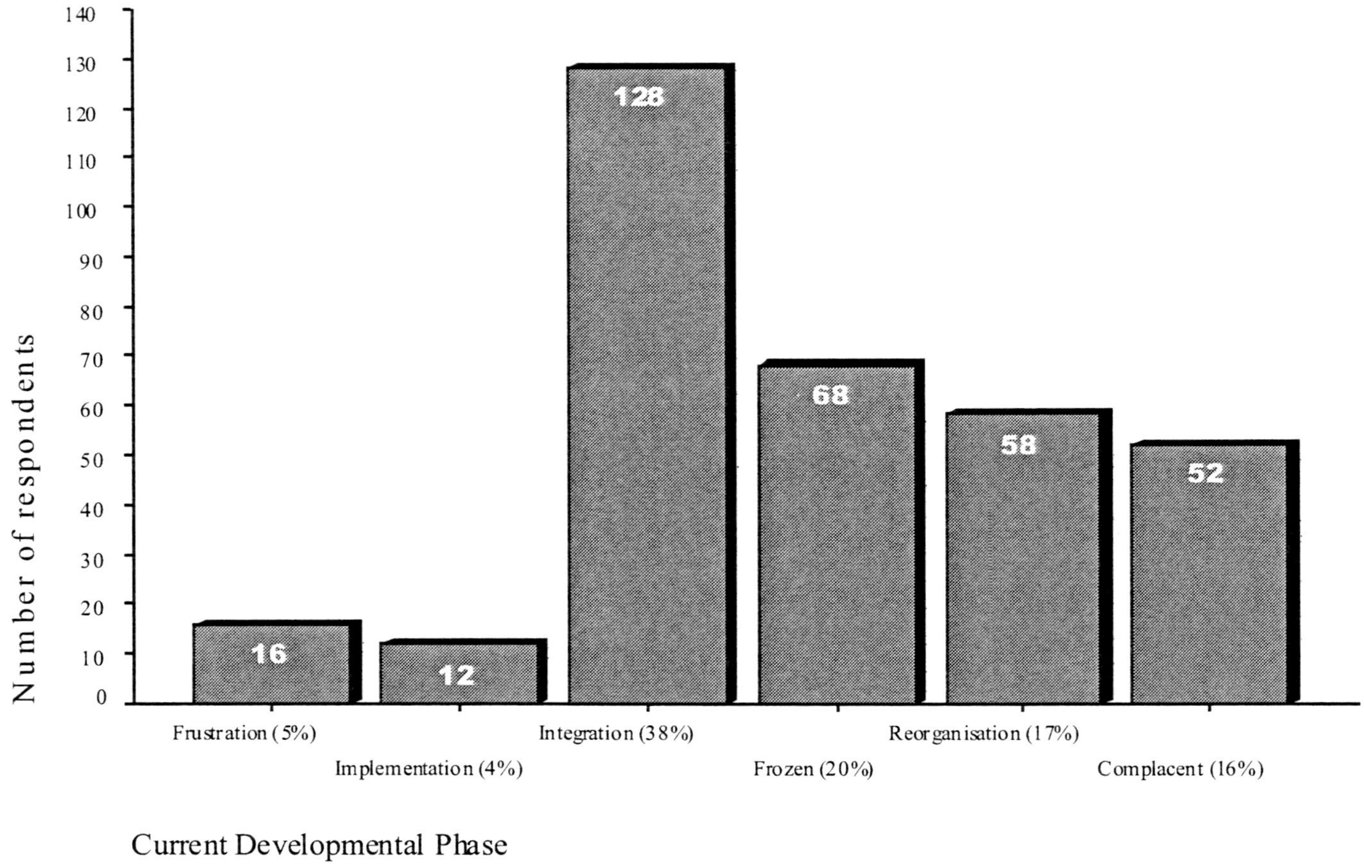

Figure 5.5 The role developmental phase which respondents were experiencing at the time of the study (N = 334)

Respondents were, in addition, asked to indicate the phase they were currently experiencing by listing it last in the above rank order of phases. No one was experiencing an orientation phase at the time of the study (*Figure 5.5*). The majority (38.3%) reported being in an integration phase, while only a small percentage were experiencing frustration (4.8%) and implementation (3.6%).

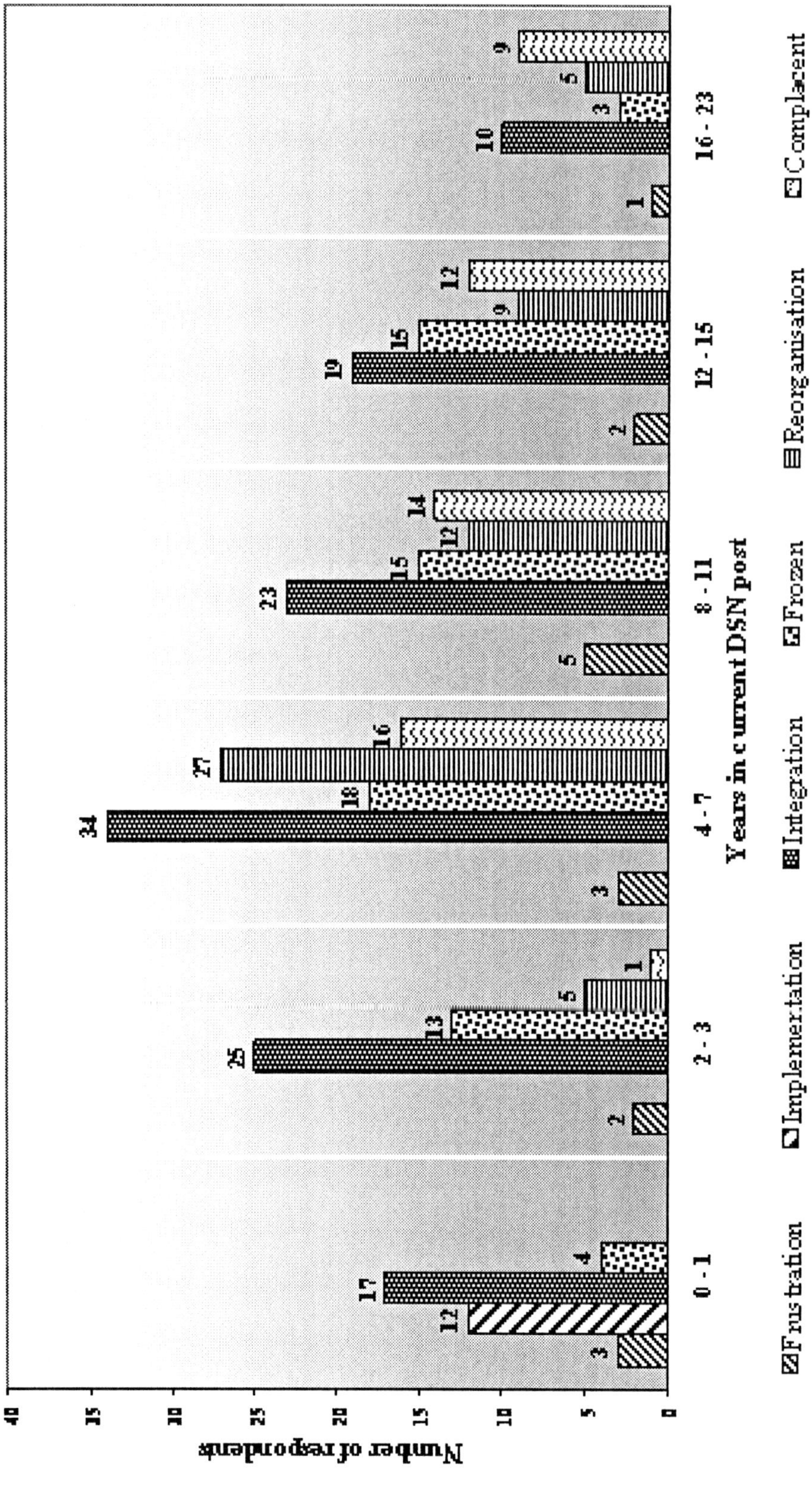

Figure 5.6 Breakdown by years of employment of developmental phases currently being experienced by respondents (N=334)

From *Figure 5.6*, which delineates a breakdown of the experience of these phases through respondents' years of employment in their DSN post, it can be seen that integration had the highest frequency among all groups. It also can be seen that frustration, integration, frozen, and reorganisation phases were present throughout all the year groups. This indicates that these phases often overlapped and, for many respondents, they did not have a particular sequence of occurrence, i.e. respondents experienced these phases at any stage of their role development. On the other hand, implementation occurred in the first year of employment, with only two respondents experiencing this phase in their second year. The complacent phase, however, occurred after the fourth year in post, apart from one DSN who reported being in this phase in the third year.

5.4.11 Facilitators and barriers to role development

At the end of this section, respondents were asked to indicate the factors that acted as facilitators and barriers to their overall role development. These and the frequency with which they were cited by respondents are listed in *Tables 5.5* and *5.6* (some respondents cited more than one facilitator and/or barrier). It can be seen that the facilitating factors identified by DSNs were similar to reasons cited earlier as contributing to positive phases. The barriers, however, were similar to reasons related to the experience of negative phases. No differences were identified in responses between novice and experienced respondents, or between respondents working in their first DSN post and those working in a second, third or fourth DSN post.

Table 5.5 Factors facilitating role development of the DSN and the frequency of their citation by respondents (N=334)

N°	Facilitating factors to role development of the DSN	Number of responses	
		Frequency	%
1	Peer support and networking with other DSNs	90	*26.9*
2	Supportive and encouraging healthcare team	38	*11.4*
3	Personal characteristics and attributes	35	*10.5*
4	Support for role by management/administration	31	*9.3*
5	Length of experience in the DSN post	30	*9.0*
6	Support and recognition of DSN role by medical staff	23	*6.9*
7	Flexibility and autonomy in role performance	23	*6.9*
8	Education/training related to diabetes care	15	*4.5*
9	Regular updates and ongoing education	13	*3.9*
10	Having a mentor/role model	12	*3.6*
11	Educational preparation at Master's level	12	*3.6*
12	Support and recognition of the DSN role by nursing staff	11	*3.3*
13	Positive feedback from patients and their families	9	*2.7*
14	Other nursing qualifications and previous experience	6	*1.8*
15	Involvement in research activities	5	*1.5*
16	Adequate facilities and resources	4	*1.2*

Table 5.6 Factors acting as barriers to role development of the DSN and the frequency of their citation by respondents (N=334)

N°	Barriers to role development of the DSN	N° of responses Frequency	%
1	Time pressures due to staff shortages and heavy workload	77	23.1
2	Lack of or constraints on resources/financial restrictions	73	21.9
3	Lack of support by management/administration	59	17.7
4	Lack of understanding of DSN role by management/health staff	38	11.4
5	Lack of role models and/or working alone with no peer support	14	4.2
6	Restraints on DSN role deriving from medical staff	14	4.2
7	Negative attitudes of other health professionals	13	3.9
8	Personal characteristics	12	3.6
9	Politics within the institution and organisational structure	12	3.6
10	Funding or time constraints for further formal education	10	3.0
11	Working within a non-supportive team (poor communication)	8	2.4
12	Inadequate space or material facilities	7	2.1
13	Lack of authority to prescribe	7	2.1
14	Limited career prospects, slow promotion	6	1.8
15	No obstacles	3	0.9

5.5 Discussion of findings and implications for practice

The *Role Development Model* by Hamric and Taylor (1989), based on experiences of CNSs in the USA, was tested in this study with DSNs working in the UK. Respondents identified similar reasons for experiencing the seven developmental phases to those reported by Hamric and Taylor. The findings suggest that similarities exist between the USA and the UK in the process of role development of specialist nurses. Moreover, this similarity indicates that the findings of the present study can be generalised not only to the overall population of DSNs, but also to other groups of CNSs.

5.5.1 Orientation phase and transition phase

According to Hamric and Taylor (1989), the orientation phase presents the first natural developmental step in learning a new role. It reflects the time required by specialist nurses to become familiar with the role and the employing organisation. The present study revealed that the experience of entrance into the role was characterised as orientation phase by respondents holding a first DSN post and as transition phase by respondents holding either a second, third or fourth DSN post. Transition phase was a new phase which emerged from the results of this study, and its characteristics have not been previously described in the literature with respect to the CNS role. This was a typical phase for experienced respondents moving into a new DSN post or changing their work setting within the same post. The term *transition*, however, has been widely used in the role theory field and has been defined as:

> *'... an event or non-event resulting in changes in individual psychosocial assumptions concerning oneself or one's organisational environment, social environment, or one's relation to one's environment.'* (Sokol and Louis, 1984: p83)

With regard to occupational roles, role transition refers to the process of moving in and out of roles, with the focus on role orientation and role performance. It may occur in a person's change of position or status, between different roles or within a role, or as a change in the content of a role (Frese, 1984).

Role transition may be associated with incongruity of the incumbent's perceptions with the demands of the new role resulting in different patterns of role stress and strain. Graduate nursing students, for example, may experience a 'reality shock' when entering employment (Kramer, 1974); this 'shock' can be extended to all professional nurses learning a new speciality. However, as Allen and van de Vliert (1984) noted, it is not necessary that role transitions have severe consequences on incumbents. They often proceed reasonably smoothly, accompanied by only a minimal degree of perturbation in the incumbent's overall psychological functioning, particularly when those transitions are towards a more desirable position or within the same role.

From the foregoing discussion, it can be concluded that both orientation and transition phases reflect a role transition process. However, it was deemed necessary to distinguish between them in order to determine the appropriate strategies used by specialist nurses in proceeding successfully through these phases. Moreover, the application of knowledge of the characteristics of these phases results in the CNS, administrators and health staff setting realistic expectations for CNS role performance.

The results of the present study showed that most DSNs who reported positive experiences of orientation phase had followed an induction programme into the role and the organisational structure of the institution. They had support and had been allowed time to feel confident and gain competence before being expected to function autonomously in the role. Experienced DSNs also cited the provision of an orientation programme as helpful at the start of their new job. However, this orientation aimed to help DSNs become familiar with the organisational structure of the work setting rather than the role itself.

According to Hamric and Taylor (1989), a structured orientation plan should be organised for newly employed CNSs whether they are novices or experienced. It should be appropriately designed to inform the CNS not only about the role itself, but also about the organisational structure, philosophy, goals, policies, and procedures of the agency (Bryckzynski, 2000). A large number of respondents in the present study identified the presence of role models and peer support as a significant factor in proceeding successfully through this phase.

Hamric (1983) suggested consensual validation and feedback must be provided by a senior CNS or a person knowledgeable in the role at least every three months for the novice CNS during the first year of employment. As Baker (1987) asserted, the first year of the CNS practice is crucial in establishing their credibility and laying the foundation for future development. Many newly qualified CNSs, guided by the theoretical knowledge of the role, often have the feeling that they should be 'everywhere at once' and 'all things to all people'. However, as Cameron (1994) points out, giving in to this urge could render the specialist nurse a physical wreck at best and a dabbler at worst. Therefore, it is particularly crucial to provide the novice CNS with help in setting limits and realistic self-expectations, in understanding how to cope with problem situations, and in maintaining a sense of perspective. The newly qualified CNS who is taught how to work within an organisation and learns who to consult for advice and guidance can then begin to develop a network for advancement and learning (Beecroft, 2001).

The experienced DSNs in this study felt very comfortable with the role and did not require a role model. They were able to undertake new projects and function autonomously as soon as they had become familiar with the new work setting. However, a number of them reported that lack of support for their role impeded their further role development. Thus it can be concluded that experience, expertise and determination are not always adequate. For an expert CNS to be able to function at full capacity, appropriate support, encouragement and recognition should be provided by the work setting.

Another important aspect to consider during the initial phase of role development is the setting of realistic expectations for the DSN entering a new post. According to Hamric and Taylor (1989), it is necessary that the CNS and the supervisor or nursing manager spend time exploring and agreeing on role expectations. It has been suggested that, during the orientation phase, novice CNSs should devote a major portion of their time to direct-care activities to substantiate their role as expert practitioners (Baker, 1987; Holt, 1987; Page and Arena, 1991; Wallymahmed, 1997). This will provide them with the competence and confidence to combine gradually other components within their practice. Moreover, the CNS who displays clinical expertise will be accepted and recognised as an expert practitioner by nursing and other healthcare staff.

A number of respondents in the present study had undertaken a diabetes course which had helped them to feel more confident when entering the post. There is a general agreement that the CNS should attend graduate education before entering the role. The purpose of this education, as Hamric and Taylor (1989: p75) state, should be to prepare graduate students for the realities of the CNS role and for the possible slowness of movement through developmental phases, especially in the first year. Previous clinical experience in the area of specialty has also been viewed as necessary before entering the CNS role. Watkinson (1997) believes that the nurses should have at least one year's experience in diabetes nursing to be granted the title of DSN. In the USA, clinical experience of one to three years is one of the requisites for entrance to the CNS graduate programmes. Hamric and Taylor stated characteristically: 'To enter a CNS position with less knowledge or skill than that of the staff nurses working within the specialty is courting failure.'

Before proceeding to the next section, it should be clarified here that the second phase described by Oda (1977) in her three-phase role development model was role transition. The ultimate goal of this phase, as Oda (1977: p375) stated, '...is to evolve a specialised nursing role that fits a specific staff and institution well.' Moreover, the CNS in this phase undertakes and is able to combine all the key-components efficiently in her practice. As seen from its definition, this phase requires the CNS to have gone through an orientation into the role and/or the new organisational setting before being able to function at this level and being recognised by others as an expert advanced practitioner.

It could be proposed that the term 'role transition' used by Oda (1977) for this phase may be misleading, as it does not conform to the definition of role transition given by role theorists (Frese, 1984; Sokol and Louis, 1984). Rather, the characteristics of this phase correspond better to those of implementation described by Hamric and Taylor (1989) and Baker (1979). Hence, although the phase that emerged from the present study and that described by Oda (1977) have the term 'transition' in common, they represent two distinct stages within the process of role development.

5.5.2 Positive phases: implementation and integration

Implementation and integration phases have been characterised by Hamric and Taylor (1989) as positive resolution of the CNS role development. This is supported by the findings of the present study. The DSNs who experienced these phases reported practising at an advanced level and were able to incorporate the key sub-roles appropriate for the particular situation with greater confidence and less stress. They reported a high level of satisfaction with themselves and their institutions, because they had seen their ideas being accomplished and had been able to influence their area of practice by undertaking new projects and effecting change. They also reported that they experienced compatibility of role expectations, as well as recognition, understanding and acceptance of their role. Health professionals and managers consulted them for different issues related to the organisation and provision of diabetes care.

The reasons identified by respondents were similar for the occurrence of both the implementation and the integration phases, although the latter phase was characterised by a higher level of practice, self-confidence, and competence. A clear distinction between the boundaries of the two phases as experienced by DSNs in this study was often difficult to define and the majority characterised these as positive phases.

On the basis of the preceding discussion, it can be asserted that the experience of implementation and integration phases reflects the successful socialisation into role of specialist nurses. According to Brim (1960), role socialisation is viewed as successful if it prepares individuals to perform adequately the roles expected of them in the course of their careers throughout society. Reasons that contributed to the occurrence of the implementation and integration phases in this study resulted from respondents' work setting and personal characteristics, as well as from the characteristics of the DSN role. However, most DSNs attributed the occurrence of positive phases, implementation and integration to the opportunity to undertake new projects and introduce improvement in their area of practice. Hamric and Taylor (1989) have suggested that a focus on one or several short-term projects is a facilitating strategy for these phases, in particular that of implementation.

During the integration phase, as the CNS has gained positive feedback and recognition relating to the effectiveness of the role, more time can be devoted to areas of scholarly interest (Page and Arena, 1991). It is important for the CNS in this phase to have a plan to guide continued role expansion and refinement over time (Brykczynski, 2000). Long-term projects and objectives should be organised and implemented. Hamric and Taylor (1989) suggest that the integrated CNS should be involved widely in research, writing and other outside professional activities and act as preceptor for graduate students.

Seeking appointment to key committees and taking part in the decision-making process are also important in broadening the organisational impact of the CNS (Brykczynski, 2000). The findings of the present study confirm this assertion. More specifically, a number of respondents attributed the experience of an integration phase to their involvement in national responsibilities relating to the organisation of diabetes care. Promotion to a higher grade or a more responsible position was also mentioned by DSNs as a facilitating factor of role development.

Other role challenges identified by respondents in the present study were related to opportunities for undertaking further academic education (funding and/or study leave from the organisation). In addition, monetary recognition is the most tangible reward for clinical excellence and, thus, it should keep pace with that of other staff of comparable education and experience within the institution (Hamric and Taylor, 1989; Oda *et al*, 1988). In the present study, almost 60% of respondents reported being dissatisfied with the salary they were getting from their job. However, in their comments DSNs did not refer to this factor and therefore it was not possible to determine whether salary had an impact on their role development.

The main factors identified by DSNs in the present study as contributing to the experience of implementation and integration phases came from their work setting. Similar factors were also reported by CNSs in the study by Hamric and Taylor (1989: p79) and included support, recognition and positive feedback from management, health professionals and patients/carers. Peer support was also seen as a significant facilitator of role development. In fact, DSNs who reported no, or limited experience of, positive phases commented that, although they had acquired an advanced level of practice, constraints resulting from their work setting impeded their further role development and expansion. Hamric and Taylor maintain that:

> *'When such circumstances arise, even the most experienced and integrated CNS needs visible administrative support and advice, as well as objective, constructive counsel from a trusted mentor.'*

5.5.3 Negative phases: frustration, frozen, reorganisation and complacent

Unlike implementation and integration, these phases share a negative and non-productive character in relation to the role development of the CNS (Brykczynski, 2000). Many respondents in the present study had experienced all the four negative phases, and the reasons associated with their occurrence were similar to those identified by CNSs in the study by Hamric and Taylor (1989). The main issue prevailing in relation to these phases was the incongruence of role expectations between respondents and other parties involved within their work setting, i.e. management, supervisors, health professionals, and patients/carers. This resulted in the occurrence of different types of role stress and the experience of role strain by respondents. Role stress, as defined by role theorists, is a consequence of difficult, conflicting, or impossible demands for occupants of different roles created by their social structure/environment. Role occupants respond to role stress with role strain, which reflects feelings generated from incongruent role expectations, such as anxiety, tension, frustration, inadequacy, depression, and reduced effectiveness (Hardy and Hardy, 1988b).

Katz and Kahn (1978) maintain that role expectations are determined by the broader organisational context. In fact, the occurrence of negative phases in both the present study and that by Hamric and Taylor (1989) was attributed mainly to factors deriving from respondents' work setting. With the exception of complacent, most respondents attributed the occurrence of negative phases to the lack of support and recognition of role by other health professionals and administration. Conflict and incongruence of role expectations or goals were reported between the above parties and respondents. Feelings engendered by respondents in these situations were characteristic of role strain and a consequence of role conflict which, as described by role theorists, refers to the

'...condition in which the focal person perceives existing role expectations as being contradictory or mutually exclusive' (Hardy and Hardy, 1988b: p203).

Characteristics of role ambiguity, which reflect the uncertainty about what the role occupant is supposed to do (Biddle, 1979; Hardy and Hardy, 1988b), were also identified in respondents' comments relating to their experience of negative phases. Lack of understanding of the DSN role by other health professionals and, in particular, by management, had resulted in lack of support and conflicting expectations. Many DSNs reported that management perceived diabetes care and their role to have a 'low profile' on their agenda. Findings of the present study support those of Hamric and Taylor (1989), where CNSs reported lack of a clear role definition in their institutions and of understanding of the potential uses of the role, particularly by administration.

The third type of role stress apparent in the present study was related to role overload: role expectations were excessive in the time available for sufficient role performance (Kahn *et al*, 1981). Time limitations due to increased workload were the second most frequently cited reason by DSNs as contributing to the occurrence of frustration and frozen phases. The increased workload was closely associated with constraints on human resources, in particular shortfall in DSN coverage, as discussed earlier in this chapter, and part-time employment. This had not allowed adequate time for respondents to consider the development and performance of the multifaceted aspects of their role; research and innovation were the most neglected sub-roles.

It has been asserted that a certain degree of role stress is inevitable in organisations and, in the short term, can be an important source of motivation (Parsons, 1966). Respondents in this study reported that the increased stress of the frustration phase was one of the main motivating forces for moving into the implementation phase. However, if uncorrected over a long-term period, role stress may be detrimental not only for role occupants (CNSs in this case), but also for individuals with whom they are in contact and collaborate within their working environment (Hardy and Hardy, 1988b).

The CNS, therefore, should engage in periodic self-assessment to recognise early signs of characteristics associated with these phases and take proactive steps to deal with the negative feelings (Brykczynski, 2000). This is even more important during the frustration phase, as CNSs have not reached an advanced level of practice and have not yet developed 'self-defence' strategies against the bureaucratic system. However, as Hamric and Taylor note, there may be times when the CNSs' supervisors or others in the work setting first become aware of their negative feelings and lack of progress. Initiation of honest and open discussion is the most important strategy in eliminating the effect of negative phases and clarifying role issues before they result into serious problems. The novice CNS is particularly vulnerable to experiencing these negative feelings and therefore needs a trusted and helpful supervisor or manager. Discussion and exchange of opinions with other CNSs who had similar experiences are helpful in relieving tension (Brykczynski, 2000; Hamric and Taylor, 1989). Monthly sessions for sharing concerns and planning future role objectives with a group of peers and supervisors/administrators facilitate movement through the frustration phase.

Time management is often a problem for many novice CNSs and, thus, they require help in reassessing priorities and setting realistic expectations for performance. Moreover, they need assistance in dealing with feelings of inadequacy and in acknowledging the slow pace of change. Hamric and Taylor (1989) suggest that novice CNSs should focus on short-term objectives that can be successfully implemented and provide evidence that staff and patients can benefit from their role. The resulting positive feedback and sense of achievement will increase their self-confidence and comfort within the role. Moreover, the development of good working relationships with team members and other health professionals, as well as establishment of self within the system, is essential in obtaining support and recognition. Continuous update and formal education to increase and maintain competence are additional strategies to move successfully through the frustration phase.

Another factor identified by respondents in the present study as contributing to the occurrence of negative phases was the lack of understanding of the nature and the potential use of their role. This, as noted earlier, resulted in lack of support, isolation and controversial dynamics within the working environment of these DSNs. As Bigbee and Amidi-Nouri (2000) state, the appointment of a CNS may be interpreted by staff as a criticism of their performance, resulting in suspicion and hostility. Christman (1991: p112) commented as follows with reference to this issue:

> *'In breaking new ground at the graduate level, the nurse specialist was perceived as a threat to the status quo because she took as her model the full professional role in its broadest sense.'*

It is, therefore, apparent that role clarification should be a priority, if not the most important objective, in the process of role development of a CNS. If others do not understand the benefits of the role, they will not support and accept specialist nurses; rather they will try to eliminate their role. A number of respondents in the present study noted the importance of having a manager with a professional background in specialist nursing. However, something like this is not always possible. Therefore, the clarification of role is a task which should be undertaken by CNSs themselves.

A strategy by which CNSs can achieve this objective is the dissemination of the role description to administration and all health professionals with whom they cooperate in their practice. This job description should be clear, understandable, well-written, and concise, but long enough to state exactly who CNSs are and what they provide in that particular setting or specialty (Cooper and Sparacino, 1990). Until the role is fully established within the organisation, CNSs should take every possible opportunity to present and clarify their role responsibilities. New CNSs should expect to be 'ambassadors' for the CNS role, explaining in a sentence or two what a CNS is and does. Furthermore, graduate educational programmes need to prepare CNS graduates to have a clear understanding of their role and to have the ability to clearly describe it to others (Hamric and Hanson, 2003).

The lower percentage of respondents in the frustration phase (5%) as compared to Hamric and Taylor's (1989) findings (13%) may be a function of the more experienced DSN respondents; only 8% were in their first year of specialist practice, compared to 16% of Hamric and Taylor's sample. The higher overall percentages of respondents in negative developmental phases (58%) as compared with Hamric and Taylor's original research (29%) may be due to a number of factors. For example, the differences in the surveys may have helped create different results. The frozen, reorganisation and complacent phases derived from respondents' comments to one open-ended question in Hamric and Taylor's study, while in the current study each phase was described. These descriptions may have resulted in more DSNs recognising negative phases in their developmental trajectory. In addition, Hamric and Taylor did their study over fifteen years ago, when the healthcare system was arguably more stable than it is today. Significant turmoil in the healthcare system could account for the greater numbers of DSNs reporting being in the reorganisation phase (17%) as compared to the CNSs in Hamric and Taylor's study (3%). Scarce resources, staff shortages and heavy workload were the main reasons for DSNs' experiences of negative phases in the present study. The higher percentage of DSNs in negative phases compared to the CNSs in Hamric and Taylor's study could also be attributed to the facts that in the UK the CNS role has not been clarified to the extent it has in the USA, and there is no nationally recognised certification for specialist nursing. Hamric and Taylor also sampled CNSs who were part of existing CNS support groups. These factors may have contributed to more CNSs being in positive developmental phases.

For the experienced CNS going through the frozen or reorganisation phases, as Hamric and Taylor (1989) state, supportive and non-judgemental counselling from an objective outsider is necessary in resolving conflict. It is important to assess whether or not the expectations or goals of the CNS are realistic, given the prevailing circumstances. When conflict develops, both the CNS and the administration or other related parties should be involved in dialogue aimed to find a satisfactory resolution of conflict. Furthermore, it is helpful for the CNS to present a written plan which provides evidence of the importance of implementing these goals by suggesting appropriate strategies for their achievement. This will provide an opportunity for active re-negotiation and realignment of role responsibilities.

A small number of DSNs in the present study reported being in a complacent phase, suggesting that the area of diabetes care and the DSN role present a lot of challenges. Similar results were also reported by Hamric and Taylor (1989). A higher percentage of DSNs were in this phase (15.6%) than CNSs in the earlier study (3%) by Hamric and Taylor (1989). This difference could be attributed to longer time within post, as almost half of respondents (N = 154) were employed as DSNs for over eight years. Most DSNs who experienced a complacent phase reported 'sit back for a while' periods of time during their career. As in frozen and reorganisation phases, the description of the complacent phase in the questionnaire could be another reason why more respondents in the current study reported experiences of this phase.

The short duration of this phase was seen as a positive and re-energising period for respondents in both studies. However, this phase was associated with negative feelings and absence of challenge for further expansion of practice by a considerable number of respondents. Hamric and Taylor (1989) contend that CNSs who remain in this phase for long periods are not seen as change agents and only meet selected, narrowly focused needs. They further suggest that the CNS should change some aspects of practice and/or focus on a new unmet need of patients or institution. Undertaking a course or formal education is another helpful strategy for moving out of this phase. Whatever the selected strategy for eliminating feelings of complacency, the employing organisation and administration should provide the greatest possible assistance to the CNS in this process.

5.6 Summary

This chapter presented the results of a large study which explored the process of role development of the DSN based on the seven role developmental phases suggested by Hamric and Taylor (1989). A new phase, the transition phase, emerged from the findings of this study. Respondents described their experiences and feelings engendered during the development of their role in terms of positive and negative phases. Positive phases maximise the potential of the CNS role performance. On the other hand, although negative experiences during role development can often be unavoidable, it is evident that CNSs should not allow themselves, nor should administrators tolerate them, remaining and practising in these negative phases. Open discussion should be initiated in order to find ways of overcoming the barriers which inhibit the successful role implementation.

However, if compromise, discussion and negotiations are unsuccessful, the administration and the CNS will find it mutually beneficial for the CNS to consider a career move. In seeking a new position, the CNS should carefully assess career goals and expectations and discuss this with the new employer, to be certain that the new job will offer challenge and satisfaction.

6

Role performance: activities and components constituting the role

6.1 Introduction

Four concepts of the CNS role theoretical framework discussed in this book were examined in a nationwide study involving 334 CNSs working in diabetes. This framework derived from role theory; the relevance of the latter to the CNS role is explored in *Chapter 2*. *Chapters 3* to *5* discussed the following concepts: personal characteristics and skills, work setting and organisational factors, and role development.

Role performance is explored in this chapter. A review of the literature regarding the activities and components constituting the CNS role is presented in the first part. The second part of the chapter discusses the development of the instrument measuring the DSN role performance. The study findings are presented and discussed in the final part. A detailed description of the study design, methods and data analysis is presented in *Chapter 3* and is mentioned only briefly in this chapter.

6.2 Role components and activities of the clinical nurse specialist

The role of the CNS is multifaceted and consists of a number of role components, competencies and activities. Different authors refer to a range of various components and activities undertaken by CNSs in their role enactment. *Table 6.1* depicts the most frequently cited components and activities of the CNS role performance since the establishment of this role in the 1970s, as identified by the literature review.

From an analysis of the frequency distribution of role components, five key components which characterise the role of the CNS prevailed with a frequency higher than 70%. These five primary role components found consistently throughout CNS practice are as follows: 1) expert practitioner (cited also as clinician or caregiver); 2) educator (teacher); 3) consultant (resource, advisor, counsellor); 4) researcher; and 5) manager (administrator, executive, leader). It is interesting to note that all authors include expert practice and education in the role of the CNS.

More specific to diabetes nursing in the UK, the Royal College of Nursing (1991) accepted the definition given by Castledine (1989) that the DSN is a nurse clinician with extended knowledge and skills in diabetes management, an educator, counsellor, manager, researcher, communicator and innovator held responsible for his or her actions. This definition, which was adopted for the purpose of this study of exploring the DSN role, besides the five basic components of the CNS role, includes the competencies of collaborator (coordinator, communicator, liaison role) and innovator (change agent). These competencies are regarded as essential components of the DSN role in the UK setting (Johns, 1997; Kyne-Grzebalski, 1997; Redmond, 1988). In addition, the majority of DSNs are either based in both hospital and community or may visit either when needed

(MacKinnon, 1998a). Therefore, collaboration is a very important aspect of the role, which enables the DSN to facilitate coordination between the two settings, as well as continuity of care.

For these reasons, the role of the DSN in this study was explored in relation to seven key components and competencies, which are discussed separately in the following part of this chapter. It should be noted that the term CNS in this book includes that of the DSN, unless the work cited refers exclusively to the role of the DSN.

Table 6.1 Role components and activities of the clinical nurse specialist role performance

	Role components / Authors	Expert practitioner, Care-giver, clinician	Teacher, educator expert coaching	Consultant, advisor, resource	Research	Administrator, leader, manager, executive	Collaborator, liaison, communicator	Innovator, change agent	Staff/patient advocate	Role model, mentor	Scholarly activities, profess. development	Quality promoter, standard setting, audit	Ethical decision-making
1	Georgopoulos & Christman (1970)	✔	✔	✔	✔	✔	✔						
2	Boucher & Bruce (1972)	✔	✔		✔			✔					
3	Gaines (1981)	✔	✔		✔			✔					
4	Castledine (1982)	✔	✔		✔		✔	✔		✔			
5	Robichaud & Hamric (1986)	✔	✔	✔	✔	✔					✔		
6	Sparacino (1986)	✔	✔	✔	✔								
7	Tarsitano *et al* (1986)	✔	✔		✔	✔							
8	Chambers *et al* (1987)	✔	✔	✔	✔	✔							
9	Menard (1987a)	✔	✔	✔	✔	✔							
10	Topham (1987)	✔	✔	✔	✔	✔							
11	RCN (1988)	✔	✔		✔	✔							
12	Redmond (1988)	✔	✔	✔	✔		✔	✔		✔		✔	
13	Ryan-Merritt *et al* (1988)	✔	✔		✔	✔	✔						
14	Storr (1988)	✔	✔	✔	✔			✔	✔				
15	Burge *et al* (1989)	✔	✔	✔							✔		
16	Castledine (1989)	✔	✔	✔	✔	✔	✔	✔					
17	Hamric & Spross (1989)	✔	✔	✔	✔	✔	✔						
18	King (1990)	✔	✔			✔		✔	✔	✔			
19	Sparacino & Cooper (1990)	✔	✔	✔	✔	✔							
20	Aikin *et al* (1993)	✔	✔	✔	✔	✔					✔		
21	Nuccio *et al* (1993)	✔	✔		✔	✔							
22	Humphris (1994a)	✔	✔	✔	✔		✔					✔	
23	McFadden & Miller (1994)	✔	✔	✔	✔	✔		✔	✔	✔	✔		
24	Miller (1995)	✔	✔	✔	✔			✔	✔				
25	Castledine *et al* (1996)	✔	✔	✔	✔	✔						✔	
26	Johns (1997)	✔	✔			✔	✔						
27	Kyne-Grzebalski (1997)	✔	✔	✔	✔	✔		✔					
28	Scott (1997)	✔	✔	✔	✔	✔							
29	McGee (1998)	✔	✔	✔	✔	✔							
30	McGee & Castledine (1998)	✔	✔	✔	✔	✔							
31	Gibson & Bamford (2001)	✔	✔	✔	✔	✔	✔						
32	Sparacino (2005)	✔	✔	✔	✔	✔	✔						✔

6.2.1 Expert practitioner

The provision of direct patient care has been a major component in the role of the CNS since its origin (Reiter, 1966). The role of the CNS was established to provide expert bedside care and thus improve the quality of patient care and nursing practice. As an expert practitioner, the CNS provides nursing care at an advanced level in his or her area of practice and demonstrates excellent clinical judgement (King, 1990; Menard, 1987b; Sparacino, 2005). Moreover, the CNS is able to develop clinical protocols for the care of patients and has the ability to manage those patients throughout the course of their condition/illness. Therefore, CNS involvement in direct care differs from that of the general nursing staff who perform the ongoing nursing activities.

Specialist care is linked to specific types of intervention for particular groups of patients experiencing unique and/or complex problems. It depends on the needs of the staff and organisation, and requires from the CNS the acquisition of more advanced skills than those of general nurses (McGee, 1998; Scott, 1997). The several stages of role development and the length of clinical experience enable the CNS to move away from rules towards a more intuitive approach in interventions, by integrating theory into practice (Benner, 2001). Clinical expertise likewise has a practical relevance when a theoretical framework for nursing practice is being developed (Sparacino, 1986). Moreover, involvement in direct care gives CNSs the opportunity to develop their practice, improve their skills, and remain informed on the latest developments.

CNSs, as expert practitioners, assess patients' condition with a high level of discriminative judgement, determine priorities of care, and plan and design with advanced knowledge and skills. Furthermore, they implement comprehensive and individualised care, and evaluate the quality of the care provided. This continuity of care assists patients/carers and complements their capacity to achieve or maintain optimum health and functioning (Koetters, 1989; Sparacino, 1986). Sparacino (2005: p421) supported the dictum that expert practice has the advantage of providing the CNS with the '...opportunity to demonstrate clinical competency, maintain clinical expertise, meet direct care requirements for recertification, identify staff learning needs, role model important clinical behaviours, evaluate resource utilization, and ensure CNS visibility and accessibility.'

The clinical expertise of the CNS should not only improve the level of care received by those patients with whom they interact, but also the overall quality of nursing care. The CNS functions as a role model for other nursing staff and as guidance in their professional career by providing expert care for patients under a theoretical orientation. However, in order to act as a role model, the CNS needs to be accepted by other members of the healthcare team as an advanced practitioner. Therefore, effective and sustained impact on clinical practice requires CNSs to prove their competence and skills as expert practitioners.

If CNSs lack such skills or are unable to translate acquired theoretical knowledge into directives for use in the practice setting realistically and comfortably, nursing staff may devalue their suggestions and even consider them as intruders (Sparacino and Cooper, 1990). Moreover, 'hands-on' practice of patient care increases the visibility of CNSs, and direct contact with patients/clients and other health professionals enables them to serve as advocates of both patients and staff. CNSs are also in a good position to evaluate nursing care and staff performance and identify appropriate means of strengthening both. Furthermore, CNSs, being involved in direct care, participate in quality assurance activities and in the setting of achievable standards of care. They are also able to generate research questions applicable to clinical practice and to identify opportunities for utilisation of research finding for evidence-based practice (Sparacino, 2005).

6.2.2 Educator

Educational responsibilities are a traditional part of the CNS role. Their practice of remaining vigilant for new, relevant information and then sharing this information in an effective and timely manner is one of their most effective teaching interventions (McCaffrey-Boyle, 1996). CNSs have a great deal of responsibility in teaching patients and their families/carers, nursing staff and other health professionals, nursing and other healthcare students, as well as the public or community (Sparacino, 2005). Thus, CNSs provide education to a wide range of people or groups. However, as McCaffrey-Boyle (1996) states, the CNS's classroom must remain the bedside, and the focus of his/her practice for the educator role component should be the patient and family.

Patient-focused instruction is the mainstay of the CNS education role and the characteristic which most differentiates it from those of staff development educators and academicians. The specialist nurse with expert knowledge and skills is in a strategic position for patient and family education, which may focus on individual or group education. Moreover, collaborative discussion of patient problems, individualised assessment, and joint decision-making are the hallmarks of conjoint patient-specific care planning and staff learning. Teaching may be structured or impromptu; it often occurs on site, but may also occur on the phone (Priest, 1989; Spross *et al*, 2000).

Part of the specialist nurse's role as an educator is to teach and inform not only patients and their families/carers, but also their colleagues, health staff and/or students. The integration of counselling and good communication skills into one-to-one exchanges with these is an effective way of conducting educational sessions and in particular when discussing difficulties. CNSs act as role models for other health professionals, by demonstrating the practical integration of theory and evidence-based practice, maintaining a focus on continuously improving clinical care, and integrating new knowledge into practice. The CNS has a professional responsibility to serve as an educator and mentor for graduate nursing students, sharing in this way their knowledge with future CNSs and demonstrating the level of advanced practice nursing to which students can aspire (Sparacino, 2005).

Development of new educational tools and programmes is another example of the CNS educational involvement. The CNS's clinical experience yields data on patients' and their families' concerns, confusion, and needs for clarification. For this reason, the CNS is in the best position to select and implement the most appropriate teaching method for each patient or situation (McCaffrey-Boyle, 1996). It is obvious that the education role component of the CNS is itself multifaceted and, therefore, requires proficiency in learning theory and practice for both professional and non-professional consumers.

6.2.3 Consultant

Consultation is the provision of assistance to enhance the consultee's ability to master a given situation. It requires availability, willingness, insight, clinical expertise, communication skills, and a non-judgemental attitude on the part of the CNS (McCaffrey-Boyle, 1996). There is considerable agreement that the consultative component of the CNS role is a highly valued role function, and that CNSs, nursing staff and, in particular, nursing administrators, view skill in the consultant role component as vitally important to the CNS effectiveness (Naylor and Brooten, 1993; Scherer *et al*, 1994; Tarsitano *et al*, 1986). The degree of importance placed on the consultative component of the CNS practice depends upon many factors. It is related to the needs of the staff and patients with whom the CNS is working, the expertise of the staff, the philosophy, goals, and priorities of nursing administration, and the goals and priorities that the CNS has established (Barron, 1989).

Effective consultation on a complex patient problem requires sensitivity. Emphasis is given to the patient's feelings and on how he or she can be assisted to accept the illness condition and adapt to a new way of living (McCaffrey-Boyle, 1996). Moreover, the CNS is a content expert and so assists in suggesting a wide range of alternative approaches or solutions to clinical or systems problems, whether internal or external to the practice setting. In addition, the CNS is a resource consultant and provides pertinent information that enables nurses and other health professionals to make decisions based on a range of relevant and appropriate alternatives (Sparacino, 2005).

The emphasis placed on the consultative role component may fluctuate over time, but nursing consultation remains an essential and valued activity for most CNSs. Likewise, consultation requests are more often informal and occur when a CNS is already present on a patient care unit, or are just as likely to be initiated in the hall or stairwell.

6.2.4 Researcher

It has been documented that the least time is spent by CNSs on implementation of the researcher role component (Humphris *et al*, 1999; Robichaud and Hamric, 1986; Scott, 1999; Tarsitano *et al*, 1986; Walker, 1986). However, the researcher role component facilitates the improvement of the quality of nursing care by scholarly inquiry and application of science to clinical practice. Research is essential to build and extend the knowledge base for nursing practice, and for greater understanding of the impact of nursing interventions on patient outcomes. Before becoming involved in research, a CNS must assess the readiness and receptiveness of the practice setting, administrative support, and whether research is a realistic performance goal at the given time (McGuire and Harwood, 2000).

Most often, the practical level of involvement is collaborative nursing and interdisciplinary research. By being a member of a research team, a CNS is in a unique position to contribute to the generation of clinically-based knowledge, to create a link between practical application and theoretical design, and to bridge the gap between how nursing ought to be and what is practised. A CNS is the clinical expert, understands the clinical issues, and has access to patients, while a nurse researcher is the research expert, knows research methodology, and has access to the resources that support the research (Sparacino, 2000). Their collaboration in undertaking a research project would undoubtedly have the desired results. Therefore, as Oddi and Cassidy (1998) propose, the absence of CNS involvement in the design and conduct of a subject-related study or the discussion of its results almost always has negative consequences. Its outcomes may be disappointing, recommendations misguided, and money misspent.

A perceptual problem that precludes CNSs from active participation in research activities is the assumption that it is only worth participating in research if one is a principal investigator. It should be emphasised that the competency of undertaking the researcher role component encompasses the continuum from scholarly inquiry to research utilisation and research conduct. Interpretation and use of research, evaluation of practice, and participation in collaborative research are three research competencies identified by Sparacino (2005) as constituting the broad spectrum of the CNS research role component.

6.2.5 Clinical and professional leadership

Clinical leadership is a major component of the CNS role and is an expectation of administrators and staff. In addition, management knowledge, skills, and processes enhance their effectiveness as clinical leaders, regardless of organisational placement. This component is integral to the role, because a CNS has responsibility for clinical innovation and change within the patient care system. The CNS has significant formal and informal impact and influence and, therefore, must be visionary yet practical. Moreover, the CNS is the link between a variety of resources and nursing staff and asserts clinical and professional leadership in the practice setting or healthcare system, in healthcare policy and delivery decisions, or in the administration of direct care programmes (Hanson and Malone, 2000; Sparacino, 2000).

Leadership is integral to the role because a CNS has responsibility for clinical innovation and change, as well as significant formal and informal impact and influence on the patient care system (Sparacino, 2005). Clinical and leadership competencies are integrated with the other CNS competencies to support the overall purpose and goals of an organisation relating to the provision of patient care. Most healthcare organisations are a bureaucratic maze. For this reason, the CNS works with staff, patients, and families to help them comprehend the complexities and wend their way through the system. Moreover, the CNS can serve as an advocate or diplomat between administrators and clinical staff, helping both groups understand the vagaries and particulars of organisational change, listening and supporting when appropriate and explaining decisions when needed (Brown, 1989).

6.2.6 Collaborator, coordinator

CNSs in their practice collaborate with nurses, physicians, other healthcare providers, and patients and their families. Therefore, they must be leaders in developing, promoting, and maintaining interdisciplinary collaboration and teamwork. Collaboration results in team building, synergism, and integrative solutions, as well as high-quality and cost-efficient patient care (Spross, 1989). According to Sparacino (2000), collaboration is an essential competency of a CNS, and it is the well-earned outcome of clinical competence, effective communication, mutual trust, valuing complementary knowledge and skills, collegiality, and a favourable organisational structure. The CNS undertakes collaboration and coordination activities when performing other role components, suggesting that the skills related to this component are vital in the integration of their role.

The outcome of CNS-coordinated collaboration is empowerment of nurses and a recognition of the nurse as a critical member of the healthcare team. Moreover, a CNS builds collaborative relationships with patients and families and provides an interface between patients, their families, and physicians. In addition, collaboration between a CNS and other healthcare professionals contributes to the expertise necessary to provide effective and efficient healthcare. The CNS can integrate the insight of many professionals with different perspectives, each providing theoretical and applied knowledge, into patient care (Hanson *et al*, 2000; Sparacino, 2005).

6.2.7 Change agent, innovator

Many authors consider that innovation overlaps all other activities and components of the CNS role, and argue that the ultimate goal of the CNS must be to succeed as change agents (Girard, 1987; Girouard, 1983; Hamric, 1989; Noone, 1987). Innovation is the most difficult role to describe, perform and/or understand, and it is not a distinct role component but rather a result that occurs as the CNS performs other role components. Lancaster (1982: p20) defined the change agent as one who:

> *'...generates ideas, introduces the innovation, develops a climate for planned change by overcoming resistance and marshalling forces for acceptance, and implements and evaluates the change.'*

Innovation refers to the ability to alter and improve something or make it different. The role of the CNS as a change agent improves patient care and nursing practice and promotes communication with other healthcare personnel. Change is a non-ending process, which, as Hanson and Malone (2000: pp284-85) state, '...must be woven into the fabric of everyday life and work.' Moreover, it is challenging and invigorating, but at the same time, can be difficult and painful.

The task of CNSs to succeed in this role component is to understand the theories of change which gives them strategies and skills to become innovative within their working environment. They should also be able to explore the dynamics of change and the culture within which it occurs (Girard, 1987). The same author concludes that, '...being a change agent is knowing that change is inevitable and perhaps, as a CNS, being able to positively influence its course' (Girard, 1987: p17).

6.3 Design and methods

6.3.1 Questionnaire design

Role theorists relate role performance to the differentiated behaviour or activities of an individual relevant to a specific position within a context which is influenced by the individual's personal characteristics, working context, and role development (Hardy and Hardy, 1988b). The purpose of this section was to explore the DSN role performance and its constituent components and activities. Moreover, it aimed to determine whether personal characteristics, work setting and role development of the DSN have an impact on their role performance. A quantitative approach, utilising a postal questionnaire, was adopted for the purpose of this study. The role performance of the DSN is composed of the following seven components and competencies: expert practice, education, consultation, management-leadership, research, collaboration, and innovation. Therefore, it was decided that the DSN role performance in this study should be examined in relation to the activities that combined each of the above seven components and competencies.

A number of studies have explored different components and activities of the CNS role (Aikin *et al*, 1993; Burge *et al*, 1989; Castledine, 1982; Gaines, 1981; McGee and Castledine, 1999; Scott, 1999; Tarsitano *et al*, 1986). However, although useful as a guide, instruments used in these studies could not be adopted for the purpose of this one, as they did not cover all the dimensions of the DSN role identified in the literature. Therefore, the design of this section was undertaken by the researcher, based on the information derived from the literature and from previous studies relevant to the topic. All possible activities identified as constituting the CNS role performance were included in this section. However, when designing the questionnaire, the researcher worded these activities in ways that reflected specifically the role of the DSN. Moreover, DSNs participating in the panel of experts reviewing the content validity of the questionnaire added further activities of their role to this section. These were not included in the literature.

A five-point Likert scale was adopted and divided into seven sub-scales, each examining a different role component. It included 62 statements (items) in the pilot study, which were reduced to 58 items in the main study questionnaire. Each statement expressed a different and unique activity undertaken by the DSN as part of his/her role. Participants were asked to indicate the frequency with which they performed each activity as they rated it on the five-point Likert scale from 1 (not at all) to 5 (very frequently). The following is an example of the instructions to participants and of items included in this section:

> *'Within the past year or so, indicate by circling a number in the appropriate column on the right how often you perform each activity that best describes your role as a Diabetes Specialist Nurse.'*

'Assess and adjust insulin dosages as required.'	1 2 3 4 5
'Plan, implement, and evaluate group teaching of patients and their families.'	1 2 3 4 5

(where, 1-not at all, 2-rarely, 3-occasionally, 4-frequently, 5-very frequently)

At the end of this section, participants were asked to indicate the percentage of total work time they spent at the time of the study in each of the following role components: expert practice, education, consultation, research, and management/leadership. The percentage of time spent in collaboration and innovation was not sought in this study, as the activities comprising these components often overlap with the above five components. Respondents were also asked to estimate the percentage of travelling time which, although not included within the DSN role description, has been proven to be an important issue in this role (Johns, 1997).

6.3.2 Validity and reliability of instrument

The initial review of the questionnaire in this study was undertaken by the researcher. As a first step, a brainstorming process was adopted by including all possible items identified in the literature relevant to the purpose of each section. A rigorous review of the content of each item was then undertaken; some items which were ambiguous were reworded or omitted, and other items which measured the same dimensions were merged. An expert in linguistics assisted the researcher in this process of content clarification and reduction of items.

Subsequently, a panel of seven experts, four researchers and three DSNs working in Northern Ireland, were invited to review the questionnaire in order to establish its content validity. After the questionnaire had been critically reviewed by experts and appropriately modified by the researcher on the basis of this review, it was pre-tested in a pilot study involving 30 DSNs working in Northern Ireland. A response rate of 63.3% (19 DSNs) was obtained and results showed a high degree of internal consistency for role performance ($\alpha = 0.95$).

6.3.3 Sample

The sampling criteria for participants in this study were nurses working in the UK full or part time in diabetes care, with children, adults, or both, and whose title was 'Diabetes Specialist Nurse' (DSN). Access to the study sample was obtained through the *Diabetes Specialist Nurse Directory 2000* (Diabetes UK, 2000), which is the most comprehensive database available. Registration in this Directory is perceived by most DSNs to be valuable to their practice. Access to the DSN group through the above database and the sample size of this study allowed for the generalisation of findings to the overall population of DSNs in the UK. Questionnaires were sent to 670 DSNs working in ten NHS executive regions of the UK. The return of the questionnaire indicated consent to participation in this study.

6.3.4 Data analysis

The 334 returned questionnaires contained valid data and were included in the analysis. The *Statistical Package for Social Sciences–Version 9.0* (SPSS-V9.0) for Windows computer program was used for this purpose. The procedure of data analysis was the same as that undertaken for the development of the Personal Characteristics and Skills Scale and the Work Setting Factors Scale. Descriptive statistics, tables and graphs were used to analyse and present the frequencies of responses. Moreover, Pearson's product-moment correlation test was used to identify any relationships between different variables. Maximum likelihood exploratory factor analysis with Promax rotation was used to explore the underlying dimensions (factors) of the items comprising the seven role components of the Role Performance Scale (a detailed description of this method is presented in *Chapter 3*). Independent samples t-test was conducted to compare the percentage of time allotted to each role component for different groups of respondents.

6.4 Results

6.4.1 Demographic details

The overall number of questionnaires returned was 341 (52.2%), of which seven were incomplete, and therefore not usable, giving a final response rate of 51.2% (334 DSNs). A proportional response rate was obtained from DSNs working in all ten NHS executive regions of the UK; a breakdown of the sample of participants from each region of the UK is presented in *Chapter 3, Table 3.1*. Eighty-nine (26.6%) respondents were working part-time as DSNs and 245 (73.4%) full-time. With regard to work setting, 97 (29.0%) respondents were based in hospital, 43 (12.9%) in the community and 194 (58.1%) were working between hospital and community.

The majority of respondents, 53.0% (177 DSNs) were employed at H grade, 36.5% (122 DSNs) at G grade, and 8.1% (27 DSNs) at I grade. Only three DSNs (0.9%) were employed at grade E and five DSNs (1.5%) at grade F. Of the 290 (86.8%) DSNs who answered the question regarding the highest academic qualification earned in nursing, 112 DSNs (39%) held a degree in nursing and 65 DSNs (22.4%) held a Master's degree. Seventy-nine per cent of the 334 respondents (264 DSNs) had undertaken (or were undertaking at the time of this survey) postgraduate training related specifically to their role as DSNs. This was mainly related to National Board Courses (ENB 928 and 998). A detailed description of the respondents' educational preparation is presented in *Chapter 3.*

6.4.2 Role performance: role components and activities

Each of the seven role components in this section was examined separately as each referred to a unique dimension of the DSN role performance. The assessment of the suitability of data for factor analysis regarding these scales (*Table 6.2*) revealed that exploratory factor analysis was an appropriate method. Similarly, the inspection of Pearson's correlation matrixes showed a large number of statistically significant inter-item correlations within each scale, but none exceeded the value of $r = 0.8$. Cronbach's coefficient alpha test indicated that all seven scales measuring role performance presented high internal consistency (*Table 6.2*).

Table 6.2 Assessment of the suitability of data for factor analysis and internal consistency levels for the seven scales measuring the DSN role performance

Role component	Determinant	KMO	Bartlett's test	Cronbach's α
Expert Practice	.0345	.756	p < .001	.646
Education	.0271	.857	p < .001	.836
Consultation	.0779	.799	p < .001	.763
Research	.0108	.882	p < .001	.883
Management/leadership	.0601	.844	p < .001	.889
Collaboration/coordination	.170	.802	p < .001	.849
Innovation	.158	.844	p < .001	.824

6.4.2.1 Expert Practice Scale

The fourteen items combined within this scale represent activities undertaken by DSNs as part of their expert practice role component (*Table 6.3*). Respondents reported undertaking most of these activities either occasionally, frequently, or very frequently (*Table 6.4*).

Table 6.3 Items combining the Expert Practice Scale within the instrument measuring the DSN role performance

Item No	Item statement for Expert Practice activities
Item 1	Collaborate with team members and other healthcare staff in assessing, planning, implementing, and evaluating comprehensive diabetes care
Item 2	Administer routine direct patient care in the field of diabetes
Item 3	Assess and adjust insulin dosages as required
Item 4	Adjust oral hypoglycaemic drugs
Item 5	Prescribe diabetes-related medications
Item 6	Order laboratory tests and diagnostic procedures
Item 7	Provide specialised direct care requiring advanced skills and knowledge to patients with complex physical problems and their families/carers
Item 8	Carry a caseload of patients with diabetes and establish long and short-term goals for care of individual patients
Item 9	Participate in interdisciplinary patient care conferences
Item 10	Provide advice and support to patients and/or their families via telephone
Item 11	Provide an out-of-hours help-line for emergency cases
Item 12	Carry out home visits to maintain follow-up in patient care
Item 13	Act as a role model for staff and students when performing direct care
Item 14	Act as a patient advocate in clinical practice

Table 6.4 Frequency with which DSNs undertook each activity within expert practice, as rated on the five-point Likert scale (N=334)

Expert practice	1		2		3		4		5		Mean	SD
	Count	%	Count	%	Count	%	Count	%	Count	%		
Item 1	-	-	-	-	43	12.9	137	41.0	154	46.1	4.33	.69
Item 2	-	-	-	-	8	2.4	51	15.3	275	82.3	4.80	.46
Item 3	-	-	-	-	-	-	39	11.7	295	88.3	4.88	.32
Item 4	57	17.1	9	2.7	40	12.0	84	25.1	144	43.1	3.75	1.46
Item 5	200	59.9	9	2.7	40	12.0	84	25.1	144	43.1	2.25	1.65
Item 6	21	6.3	23	6.9	66	19.8	110	32.9	114	34.1	3.82	1.16
Item 7	-	-	-	-	48	14.4	124	37.1	162	48.5	4.34	.72
Item 8	-	-	-	-	11	3.3	58	17.4	265	79.3	4.76	.50
Item 9	-	-	54	16.2	126	37.7	84	25.1	70	21.0	3.51	.99
Item 10	-	-	-	-	-	-	30	9.0	304	91.0	4.91	.29
Item 11	140	41.9	45	13.5	51	15.3	26	7.8	72	21.6	2.54	1.59
Item 12	39	11.7	21	6.3	58	17.4	76	22.8	140	41.9	3.77	1.36
Item 13	-	-	-	-	44	13.2	136	40.7	154	46.1	4.33	.70
Item 14	-	-	-	-	45	13.5	120	35.9	169	50.9	4.37	.71

1-not at all, 2-rarely, 3-occasionally, 4-frequently, 5-very frequently

The fourteen items of this scale were subjected to an exploratory factor analysis where Kaiser's criterion suggested a four-factor solution. However, as the mean communality for this scale was 0.579, three factors were retained on the basis of Cattell's scree-plot test. The three-factor model explained 38% of the total variance. The three factors were interpreted based on an examination of the content of the items loading on each factor (*Table 6.5*). A moderate correlation was found between Factors 1 and 2 ($r = 0.419$; $p < 0.01$), as well as between Factors 2 and 3 ($r = 0.306$; $p < 0.01$). A low correlation was found between Factors 1 and 3 ($r = 0.191$; $p < 0.01$), suggesting a differentiation in the performance of direct care and advanced specialised care activities by DSNs. An examination of the content of the items which loaded on each of the three factors (*Table 6.5*) gave the following theoretical interpretation for each factor.

Table 6.5 Item loadings on each of the three factors of the Expert Practice Scale

Pattern Matrix[a]

		Factor		
		1	2	3
Item 2	Expert Practice	*.910*		
Item 10	Expert Practice	*.662*		
Item 8	Expert Practice	*.644*		
Item 3	Expert Practice	*.506*		
Item 14	Expert Practice		*.718*	
Item 13	Expert Practice		*.652*	
Item 12	Expert Practice		*.428*	*-.328*
Item 11	Expert Practice		*.422*	
Item 9	Expert Practice		*.415*	
Item 1	Expert Practice		*.316*	
Item 4	Expert Practice			*.704*
Item 6	Expert Practice			*.644*
Item 7	Expert Practice			*.549*
Item 5	Expert Practice			*.480*

Extraction Method: Maximum Likelihood
Rotation Method: Promax with Kaiser Normalisation

[a]. 1-Direct care; 2-Liaison and indirect care; 3-Advanced specialised care

6.4.2.1.1 Factor 1: Direct care

This factor described the routine direct care activities undertaken by respondents in the performance of their role as expert practitioners and included four items (*Table 6.5*). The activities that correspond to these items are described in *Table 6.3*. The highest loading (0.910) was reported for Item 2, 'Administer routine direct patient care in the field of diabetes', the content of which bears a close resemblance to the title of this factor. It accounted for 83% of the variance explained by this factor. Cronbach's alpha coefficient test suggested that the dimensions of this factor present a reliable measure of direct care activities ($\alpha = 0.767$).

6.4.2.1.2 Factor 2: Liaison and indirect care

As seen in *Table 6.5*, six items loaded on this factor (refer to *Table 6.3* for a description of activities represented by these items). These items refer to liaison and indirect care activities undertaken by DSNs as part of their expert practice role component. The highest loading (0.718) was recorded for Item 14, 'Act as patient advocate in clinical practice', indicating that 52% of the variance was accounted for by this factor. Cronbach's alpha test indicated that the dimensions of this factor present a reliable measure of liaison and indirect care activities undertaken by the DSN as part of expert practice ($\alpha = 0.608$).

6.4.2.1.3 Factor 3: Advanced specialised care

Four items, the description of which can be seen in *Table 6.3*, loaded on this factor which represents specialised activities undertaken by DSNs requiring advanced knowledge and skills (*Table 6.5*). The highest loading (0.704) was recorded for Item 4, 'Adjust oral hypoglycaemic drugs', which accounted for 50% of the variance explained by this factor.

The majority of respondents reported undertaking advanced specialised care either occasionally or frequently (Mean = 3.54; SD = 0.90). An exception was Item 5, suggesting that almost 60% of respondents did not prescribe any diabetes-related medications (*Table 6.4*). Most of the remaining 40%, however, commented that they were involved in this activity in the following forms: prescribing blood glucose strips, lancets and syringes; recommending treatment types and doses to medical colleagues; and/or filling in prescription forms for GPs and/or hospital doctors to sign.

In addition, 57 (17.1%) respondents reported not being involved in the adjustment of oral hypoglycaemic drugs. However, from a cross-tabulation of responses, it was found that 49 of these 57 respondents were paediatric DSNs. Cronbach's alpha test indicated that the dimensions of this factor present a reliable measure of advanced specialised care activities undertaken by the DSN ($\alpha = 0.646$).

6.4.2.2 Education Scale

The ten items combined within this scale represent activities undertaken by DSNs as part of their education role component (*Table 6.6*). The majority of respondents in this study reported undertaking all the indicated teaching activities, with a frequency that varied from occasionally to very frequently (*Table 6.7*).

Table 6.6 Items combining the Education Scale within the instrument measuring the DSN role performance

Item No	Item statement for education activities
Item 1	Coordinate and/or participate in the education and training of nursing staff
Item 2	Provide education to medical staff
Item 3	Contribute to the educational and professional development of nursing and/or other healthcare students
Item 4	Develop/participate in the development, implementation, and/or evaluation of educational resources and materials that facilitate diabetes education
Item 5	Plan, initiate and evaluate individual patient teaching programmes
Item 6	Plan, implement, and evaluate group teaching of patients and their families
Item 7	Coordinate and/or participate in community and public educational and informational programmes
Item 8	Take part in the delivery of formal academic education in diabetes
Item 9	Organise, in collaboration with other members of the healthcare team, seminars on diabetes and workshops for healthcare professionals
Item 10	Provide diabetes education to people who are in contact with the person with diabetes, such as school teachers, employers, friends

Table 6.7 Frequency with which DSNs undertook each activity within education, as rated on the five-point Likert scale (N=334)

Education	1		2		3		4		5		Mean	SD
Item No	Coun	%	Count	%	Count	%	Count	%	Count	%		
Item 1	-	-	-	-	41	12.3	145	43.4	148	44.3	4.32	.68
Item 2	12	3.6	38	11.4	143	42.8	83	24.9	58	17.4	3.41	1.02
Item 3	-	-	7	2.1	69	20.7	150	44.9	108	32.3	4.07	.78
Item 4	-	-	22	6.6	85	25.4	133	39.8	94	28.1	3.90	.89
Item 5	-	-	11	3.3	46	13.8	138	41.3	139	41.6	4.21	.80
Item 6	27	8.1	34	10.2	70	21.0	95	28.4	108	32.3	3.67	1.25
Item 7	9	2.7	48	14.4	125	37.4	94	28.1	58	17.4	3.43	1.02
Item 8	34	10.2	36	10.8	109	32.6	107	32.0	48	14.4	3.30	1.15
Item 9	10	3.0	26	7.8	111	33.2	134	40.1	53	15.9	3.58	.95
Item 10	11	3.3	36	10.8	121	36.2	88	26.3	78	23.4	3.56	1.06

1-not at all, 2-rarely, 3-occasionally, 4-frequently, 5-very frequently

Two factors were extracted based on Cattell's scree-test criterion, which explained the underlying dimensions of the Education Scale. The two factors (*Table 6.8*), which explained 45% of the total variance, presented a high correlation ($r = 0.641$; $p < 0.001$), indicating the close association between the dimensions of this role component.

6.4.2.2.1 *Factor 1: Educating health staff*

The five items of this factor (*Table 6.8*) described the education provided by respondents to other health professionals relating to diabetes topics (refer to *Table 6.6* for a description of the activities represented by these items). The highest loading (0.807) was recorded for Item 1, 'Coordinate and/or participate in the education and training of nursing staff', indicating that 65% of the variance was accounted for by this factor. As indicated by the mean score of items constituting this factor, most respondents provided education to health professionals and students either frequently or occasionally (Mean = 3.74; SD = 0.70) (*Table 6.7*). Cronbach's alpha test revealed that the dimensions of this factor presented a high level of internal consistency ($\alpha = 0.813$).

6.4.2.2.2 *Factor 2: Educating patients, families and the public*

Five items loaded on this factor (*Table 6.8*) which reflects DSN education for people with diabetes and their families/carers, as well as the public. The detailed description of the activities represented by these items is given in *Table 6.6*. The highest loading (0.709) on this factor was recorded for Item 4, explaining 50% of the variance. This item referred to the development and implementation of educational resources and materials that facilitate diabetes education. More than 93% of respondents reported undertaking this activity at a frequency higher than 'Occasionally' (*Table 6.7*).

In general, most respondents provided education to patients, their families or carers and public with a frequency which varied from occasionally to very frequently (Mean = 3.75; SD = 0.71). The dimensions of this factor presented a high internal consistency ($\alpha = 0.737$).

Table 6.8 Item loadings on each of the two factors of the Education Scale

Pattern Matrix[a]

		Factor	
		1	2
Item 1	Education	*.807*	
Item 8	Education	*.790*	
Item 9	Education	*.700*	
Item 3	Education	*.587*	
Item 2	Education	*.545*	
Item 4	Education		*.709*
Item 5	Education		*.701*
Item 6	Education		*.670*
Item 10	Education		*.411*
Item 7	Education		*.317*

Extraction method: Maximum likelihood

Rotation method: Promax with Kaiser normalisation

[a] 1-Educating health staff

2-Educating patients, families and public

6.4.2.3 Consultation Scale

Nine items which represent activities undertaken by DSNs as part of their consultation role were included in this scale (*Table 6.9*). As presented in *Table 6.10*, a wide range of responses was received, with the majority of respondents undertaking these activities either occasionally or frequently. The exception was Item 9, with more than 70% of respondents providing consultation for patients and their families very frequently.

On the other hand, more than 50% did not participate in setting standards of diabetes care at a national level (Item 4). Despite this, the fact that 26 (7.8%) respondents were involved in this activity either frequently or very frequently makes this a significant finding. It indicates that the influence of the DSN in the organisation of diabetes care extends to national level.

Table 6.9 Items combining the Consultation Scale within the instrument measuring the DSN role performance

Item N°	Item statement for Consultation activities
Item 1	Consult with nurse managers/ward sisters to identify clinical activities that facilitate the professional growth of the nursing staff
Item 2	Provide leadership in the assessment, development, and/or implementation of policies, protocols, procedures, and care pathways in my area of practice
Item 3	Participate in setting, and/or implementing standards and targets of diabetes care in my area of practice and/or health board (district, trust)
Item 4	Participate in setting standards of diabetes care at a national level
Item 5	Facilitate the organisation of patient support group(s) in my area of practice or health board (district, trust)
Item 6	Act as a resource person for staff and students in the area of diabetes care
Item 7	Function on an 'on-call' basis for nursing and/or staff who need assistance in solving complex problems related to diabetes care
Item 8	Provide answers to clinical problems identified by healthcare personnel or try/know where to find the answers when not available
Item 9	Help patients with diabetes and their families/carers to cope with the immediate crisis of diagnosis and long-term adjustments in life style

Table 6.10 Frequency with which DSNs undertook each activity within consultation, as rated on the five-point Likert Scale (N=334)

Consultation	1		2		3		4		5		Mean	SD
Item No	Count	%	Count	%	Count	%	Count	%	Count	%		
Item 1	20	6.0	54	16.2	134	40.1	93	27.8	33	9.9	3.19	1.02
Item 2	9	2.7	31	9.3	105	31.4	140	41.9	49	14.7	3.57	.94
Item 3	15	4.5	55	16.5	96	28.7	129	38.6	39	11.7	3.37	1.03
Item 4	173	51.8	91	27.2	44	13.2	20	6.0	6	1.8	1.79	1.01
Item 5	92	27.5	85	25.4	88	26.3	48	14.4	21	6.3	2.46	1.21
Item 6	-	-	10	3.0	33	9.9	148	44.3	143	42.8	4.27	.76
Item 7	81	24.3	36	10.8	59	17.7	95	28.4	63	18.9	3.07	1.46
Item 8	-	-	14	4.2	60	18.0	165	49.4	95	28.4	4.02	.80
Item 9	-	-	-	-	13	3.9	87	26.0	234	70.1	4.66	.55
1-not at all, 2-rarely, 3-occasionally, 4-frequently, 5-very frequently												

Both Kaiser's eigenvalues and Cattell's scree-plot criteria suggested a two-factor solution for the Consultation Scale, which explained 41% of the total variance. A high correlation was found between these factors ($r = 0.532$; $p < 0.001$), indicating a close association between their dimensions. The examination of the content of the items that loaded on each of the two factors (*Table 6.11*) gave the theoretical interpretation for each factor shown in *Table 6.11*.

Table 6.11 Item loadings on each of the two factors of the Consultation Scale

Pattern Matrix[a]

		Factor	
		1	2
Item 2	Consultation	*.879*	
Item 3	Consultation	*.820*	
Item 1	Consultation	*.645*	
Item 4	Consultation	*.512*	
Item 5	Consultation	*.470*	
Item 8	Consultation		*.703*
Item 9	Consultation		*.590*
Item 6	Consultation		*.534*
Item 7	Consultation		*.387*

Extraction method: Maximum likelihood

Rotation method: Promax with Kaiser normalisation

a. 1-Consultation regarding the organisation of care

2-Consultation for health staff, patients and families

6.4.2.3.1 Factor 1: Consultation regarding the organisation of care

This factor (*Table 6.11*) described consultation activities undertaken by respondents regarding the organisation of diabetes care, and included five items (refer to *Table 6.9* for a description of activities represented by these items). The highest loadings (0.879 and 0.820) were recorded for Items 2 and 3, which accounted for 77% and 67% respectively of the variance explained by this factor. These items referred to respondents' participation in and consultation with regard to the organisation of diabetes care in their area of practice and/or health district. The mean obtained from the scores of items constituting this factor indicate that most respondents provided consultation with respect to the organisation of care occasionally (Mean = 2.88; SD = 0.78) (*Table 6.10*). The dimensions of this factor present a highly reliable measure of the DSN consultation activities in the organisation of diabetes care ($\alpha = 0.795$).

6.4.2.3.2 Factor 2: Consultation for health staff, patients and families

Four items, the description of which is presented in *Table 6.9*, loaded on this factor (*Table 6.11*). They reflect consultation activities undertaken by DSNs for health staff, as well as patients and their families/carers. The highest loading was found for Item 8 (0.703), indicating that 49% of the total variance was accounted for by this factor. This item reflected the ability of DSNs to provide answers to clinical problems related to their area of practice and identified by health professionals. Almost 80% of respondents reported providing this type of consultation either frequently or very frequently (*Table 6.10*). The majority of respondents provided consultation for health staff, patients and families either frequently or very frequently (Mean = 4.01; SD = 0.62). Cronbach's alpha coefficient test revealed a moderate internal consistency of the dimensions of this factor ($\alpha = 0.548$).

6.4.2.4 Research Scale

The eleven items combined within this scale represent activities undertaken by DSNs as part of their research role component (*Table 6.12*). Descriptive statistics presented in *Table 6.13* show that, although a wide range of responses was received, most respondents rated the frequency of their involvement in research with 'not at all', 'rarely' or 'occasionally'. Research activities which respondents were mostly involved in were related to their participation in product evaluation (Item 7) and in patient outcome evaluations (Item 11).

Table 6.12 Items combining the Research Scale within the instrument measuring the DSN role performance

Item No	Item statement for research activities
Item 1	Identify nursing care problems and develop relevant questions for systematic study
Item 2	Conduct research related to diabetes and/or other areas of nursing practice
Item 3	Communicate own research findings through presentations or publications
Item 4	Disseminate own and/or other research findings to staff, and suggest appropriate means of implementing these in practice
Item 5	Participate in a nursing research committee(s)
Item 6	Collaborate with other healthcare professionals in research
Item 7	Participate in product evaluation
Item 8	Develop proposals for funding nursing research
Item 9	Contribute to the nursing literature through publications
Item 10	Act as a preceptor and resource for staff and/or students conducting research
Item 11	Develop and conduct patient outcome evaluations

Table 6.13 Frequency with which DSNs undertook each activity within research, as rated on the five-point Likert scale (N=334)

Research	1		2		3		4		5		Mean	SD
Item No	Count	%	Count	%	Count	%	Count	%	Count	%		
Item 1	55	*16.5*	94	*28.1*	109	*32.6*	61	*18.3*	15	*4.5*	*2.66*	*1.09*
Item 2	74	*22.2*	102	*30.5*	112	*33.5*	33	*9.9*	13	*3.9*	*2.43*	*1.06*
Item 3	117	*35.0*	93	*27.8*	84	*25.1*	32	*9.6*	8	*2.4*	*2.16*	*1.08*
Item 4	66	*19.8*	71	*21.3*	109	*32.6*	76	*22.8*	12	*3.6*	*2.69*	*1.13*
Item 5	210	*62.9*	75	*22.5*	35	*10.5*	11	*3.3*	3	*.9*	*1.56*	*.87*
Item 6	56	*16.8*	99	*29.6*	107	*32.0*	61	*18.3*	11	*3.3*	*2.62*	*1.07*
Item 7	26	*7.8*	63	*18.0*	147	*44.0*	75	*22.5*	23	*6.9*	*3.02*	*1.00*
Item 8	212	*63.5*	81	*24.3*	33	*9.9*	8	*2.4*	-	-	*1.51*	*.77*
Item 9	167	*50.0*	90	*26.9*	56	*16.8*	13	*3.9*	8	*2.4*	*1.82*	*1.00*
Item 10	82	*24.6*	74	*22.2*	120	*35.9*	45	*13.5*	13	*3.9*	*2.50*	*1.12*
Item 11	85	*25.4*	67	*20.1*	119	*35.6*	52	*15.6*	11	*3.3*	*2.51*	*1.13*

1-not at all, 2-rarely, 3-occasionally, 4-frequently, 5-very frequently

A one-factor solution was reached for this scale, which explained 41% of the total variance. All the eleven items of the research scale loaded substantially (higher than 0.3) on this factor (*Table 6.14*). The percentage of variance which was accounted for by this factor ranged from 61% for Item 3, 'Communicate own research findings through presentations or publications' (loading = 0.780) to 28% for Item 9, 'Contribute to the nursing literature through publications' (loading = 0.531).

Table 6.14 Item loadings on the research factor

Pattern Matrix[a]

		Factor
		1
Item 3	Research	.780
Item 2	Research	.734
Item 4	Research	.726
Item 1	Research	.669
Item 11	Research	.657
Item 6	Research	.640
Item 8	Research	.584
Item 10	Research	.581
Item 7	Research	.544
Item 5	Research	.544
Item 9	Research	.531

Extraction method: Maximum likelihood

[a]. 1-Factors extracted; 5-iterations required

6.4.2.5 Management/leadership scale

Five items which represent activities undertaken by DSNs as part of their role as managers and leaders constituted this scale (*Table 6.15*). A wide range of responses was received relating to the frequency with which respondents undertook each of these activities as rated on the five-point Likert scale (*Table 6.16*). However, as seen from the mean scores of each item, most respondents were either not involved or were rarely involved in management and leadership activities. An exception was Item 5, indicating that almost half of respondents participated either frequently or very frequently in identifying gaps in diabetes care services.

Table 6.15 Items combining the Management/leadership Scale within the instrument measuring the DSN role performance

Item No	Item statement for Management/leadership activities
Item 1	Participate in financial and budget planning for the diabetes specialty area
Item 2	Represent nursing administration in the review of policies and procedures of departmental and/or institutional committees
Item 3	Perform or provide input into staff evaluations
Item 4	Participate in decisions regarding employment of nursing personnel
Item 5	Participate in identifying gaps in the diabetes care services

Table 6.16 Frequency with which DSNs undertook each activity within management/leadership, as rated on the five-point Likert scale (N=334)

Manag/nt	1		2		3		4		5		Mean	SD
Item No	Count	%	Count	%	Count	%	Count	%	Count	%		
Item 1	175	52.4	59	17.7	44	13.2	33	9.9	23	6.9	2.01	1.29
Item 2	114	34.1	77	23.1	77	23.1	39	11.7	27	8.1	2.37	1.28
Item 3	116	34.7	59	17.7	76	22.8	58	17.4	25	7.5	2.45	1.32
Item 4	98	29.3	72	21.6	83	24.9	46	13.8	35	10.5	2.54	1.32
Item 5	16	4.8	46	13.8	114	34.1	110	32.9	48	14.4	3.38	1.04

1-not at all, 2-rarely, 3-occasionally, 4-frequently, 5-very frequently

As in the research scale, a one-factor solution was obtained for this scale which explained 62% of the total variance. All five items in this scale presented very high loadings on this factor (*Table 6.17*), with the highest recorded for Item 3, 'Perform or provide input into staff evaluations', explaining 73% of the variance.

The relationship between management activities and respondents' employment grade was investigated using Pearson's r correlation coefficient test. A high positive correlation ($r = 0.453$; $p < 0.001$) was found, indicating that respondents holding a higher grade were more frequently involved in management activities.

Table 6.17 Item loadings on the management/leadership factor

Pattern Matrix[a]

		Factor 1
Item 3	Management/leadership	.856
Item 2	Management/leadership	.817
Item 4	Management/leadership	.816
Item 1	Management/leadership	.745
Item 5	Management/leadership	.690

Extraction method: Maximum likelihood

[a] 1-Factors extracted; 5-iterations required

6.4.2.6 Collaboration/coordination scale

Four items were included in this scale which examined the role of the DSN as collaborator and coordinator of the organisation of diabetes care (*Table 6.18*). Although a wide variety of responses was received relating to these activities, a high degree of involvement was reported by most respondents in the present study. As seen in *Table 6.19*, more than 75% of respondents were undertaking most collaboration activities either frequently or very frequently. The one-factor solution obtained for this scale explained 60% of the total variance. As seen in *Table 6.20*, all four items of this scale loaded very highly on this factor.

Table 6.18 Items combining the Collaboration/coordination Scale within the instrument measuring the DSN role performance

Item No	Item statement for Collaboration/coordination activities
Item 1	Communicate and interpret nursing assessment of people with diabetes to medical staff and other relevant healthcare personnel
Item 2	Coordinate and facilitate transfer or discharge planning between different care settings (primary-secondary-tertiary care) and/or departments
Item 3	Initiate, direct, and/or facilitate patient referrals to appropriate healthcare professionals and/or community resources or agencies
Item 4	Utilise and coordinate the varied resources and facilities for diabetes care in my area of practice

Table 6.19 Frequency with which DSNs undertook each activity included within collaboration/coordination, as rated on the five-point Likert Scale (N=334)

Collab/on	1		2		3		4		5		Mean	SD
Item No	Count	%	Count	%	Count	%	Count	%	Count	%		
Item 1	-	-	12	*3.6*	43	*12.9*	153	*45.8*	126	*37.7*	*4.18*	*.79*
Item 2	12	*3.6*	28	*8.4*	80	*24.0*	128	*38.3*	86	*25.7*	*3.74*	*1.05*
Item 3	-	-	19	*5.7*	64	*19.2*	147	*44.0*	104	*31.1*	*4.01*	*.86*
Item 4	-	-	26	*7.8*	63	*18.9*	150	*44.9*	95	*28.4*	*3.94*	*.89*

1-not at all, 2-rarely, 3-occasionally, 4-frequently, 5-very frequently

Table 6.20 Item loadings on the collaboration/coordination factor

Pattern Matrix[a]

		Factor
		1
Item 3	Collaboration/co-ordination	*.856*
Item 2	Collaboration/co-ordination	*.817*
Item 4	Collaboration/co-ordination	*.816*
Item 1	Collaboration/co-ordination	*.745*

Extraction method: Maximum likelihood

a. 1-Factors extracted; 5-iterations required

In the expert practice scale two items, 1 and 9, described activities related to DSNs' collaborative working with other health professionals in the organisation of diabetes care (*Table 6.3*). The relationship between the mean score of these items and the collaboration/coordination scale was examined using Pearson's correlation test. A moderate sig nificant correlation ($r = 0.287$, $p < 0.001$) was found, indicating that, although these activities are similar, they measure distinct dimensions of the DSN role.

6.4.2.7 Innovation scale

Five items which represent activities undertaken by DSNs as part of their role as innovators and change agents constituted the last scale in the instrument measuring the DSN role performance (*Table 6.21*). A wide range of responses was received relating to the frequency with which respondents undertook each of these activities as rated on the five-point Likert scale (*Table 6.22*). However, the majority of respondents undertook innovation activities at a frequency which varied from occasionally to very frequently.

Table 6.21 Items combining the Innovation Scale within the instrument measuring the DSN role performance

Item No	Item statement for innovation activities
Item 1	Implement in practice recent innovations and research findings related to diabetes care and evaluate their impact on the quality of care
Item 2	Implement and evaluate appropriate nursing models in the care of people with diabetes and their families/carers
Item 3	Identify, implement, and evaluate in collaboration with healthcare staff new ways of improving diabetes care
Item 4	Design presentations for the administrative authority, outlining needs for change and feasible steps for realising the goals
Item 5	Continuously monitor changing needs of diabetes care, and institute/facilitate appropriate change

Table 6.22 Frequency with which DSNs undertook each activity within innovation, as rated on the five-point Likert scale (N=334)

Innovation	1		2		3		4		5		Mean	SD
Item No	Count	%	Count	%	Count	%	Count	%	Count	%		
Item 1	12	3.6	25	7.5	90	26.9	158	47.3	49	14.7	3.62	.95
Item 2	38	11.4	51	15.3	125	37.4	93	27.8	27	8.1	3.06	1.10
Item 3	-	-	19	5.7	92	27.5	171	51.2	52	15.6	3.77	.78
Item 4	73	21.9	71	2.3	109	32.6	61	18.3	20	6.0	2.65	1.18
Item 5	-	-	33	9.9	108	32.3	145	43.4	48	14.4	3.62	.85

1-not at all, 2-rarely, 3-occasionally, 4-frequently, 5-very frequently

The one-factor solution explained 51% of the total variance in the innovation scale and all the five items of this scale loaded highly on this factor (*Table 6.23*).

Table 6.23 Item loadings on the innovation factor

Pattern Matrix[a]

		Factor
		1
Item 3	Innovation/change agent	*.784*
Item 1	Innovation/change agent	*.757*
Item 2	Innovation/change agent	*.756*
Item 5	Innovation/change agent	*.644*
Item 4	Innovation/change agent	*.601*

Extraction method: Maximum likelihood

[a] 1-Factors extracted; 5-iterations required

6.4.3 Correlations between role components

The relationship between the seven role components (as measured by the respective scale for each component) was investigated using Pearson's product-moment correlation test. The means of those components, which involved more than one factor, were included in the analysis. As seen in *Table 6.24*, all the components correlated with each other at the $p < 0.001$ level of significance, supporting the assertion that their constituent activities interconnect and may overlap.

The highest correlation was found between education and consultation ($r = 0.662$; $p < 0.001$), indicating a close association between their constituent activities. In fact, consultation correlated highly with most of the role components in this study, suggesting that DSNs undertake consultation simultaneously with activities included in other role components. A high correlation was also found between research and innovation ($r = 0.557$; $p < 0.001$), denoting that achievement of change is in close relationship to participation in research activities.

Table 6.24 Examination of the relationships between components constituting the DSN role performance using Pearson's correlation coefficient r test (N=334)

Expert Practice	Pearson r Sig. p	*1.000* .						
Education	Pearson r Sig. p	*.513**** *.000*	*1.000* .					
Consultation	Pearson r Sig. p	*.480**** *.000*	*.662**** *.000*	*1.000* .				
Research	Pearson r Sig. p	*.304**** *.000*	*.503**** *.000*	*.587**** *.000*	*1.000* .			
Management/ leadership	Pearson r Sig. p	*.241**** *.000*	*.303**** *.000*	*.496**** *.000*	*.460**** *.000*	*1.000* .		
Collaboration/ coordination	Pearson r Sig. p	*.376**** *.000*	*.445**** *.000*	*.526**** *.000*	*.329**** *.000*	*.339**** *.000*	*1.000* .	
Innovation	Pearson r Sig. p	*.322**** *.000*	*.500**** *.000*	*.618**** *.000*	*.557**** *.000*	*.507**** *.000*	*.479**** *.000*	*1.000* .
Role Component		Expert practice	Education	Cons/ion	Research	Man/ment lead/ship	Coll/tion coord/ion	Inno/tion

***Correlation is significant at the 0.01 level (2-tailed)

6.4.4 Time allotted to role components and activities

Respondents were asked to indicate the time they allotted to each of the following role components: expert practice, education, consultation, research, and management. The percentage of time that respondents spent travelling between one location and another was also sought.

As delineated in *Figure 6.1*, the majority of respondents in this study spent the greatest percentage of their total working time in expert practice activities. This percentage varied from 10% to 80% (Mean = 42.6%; SD = 16.4). The second greatest percentage after expert practice related to education, which varied from 5% to 60% (Mean = 23.8%; SD = 10.2). Furthermore, the percentage of time allotted to consultation varied from 0 to 50% (Mean = 14.7%; SD = 8.3), while for management it also varied from 0% to 50%, but the mean time was smaller (Mean = 8.7%; SD = 9.7). Respondents in this study spent the least time in research activities, varying from 0 to 40% (Mean = 4.2%; SD = 4.9). Finally, the percentage of total work time that respondents spent in travelling varied from 0 to 20% (Mean = 6.1%; SD = 4.5).

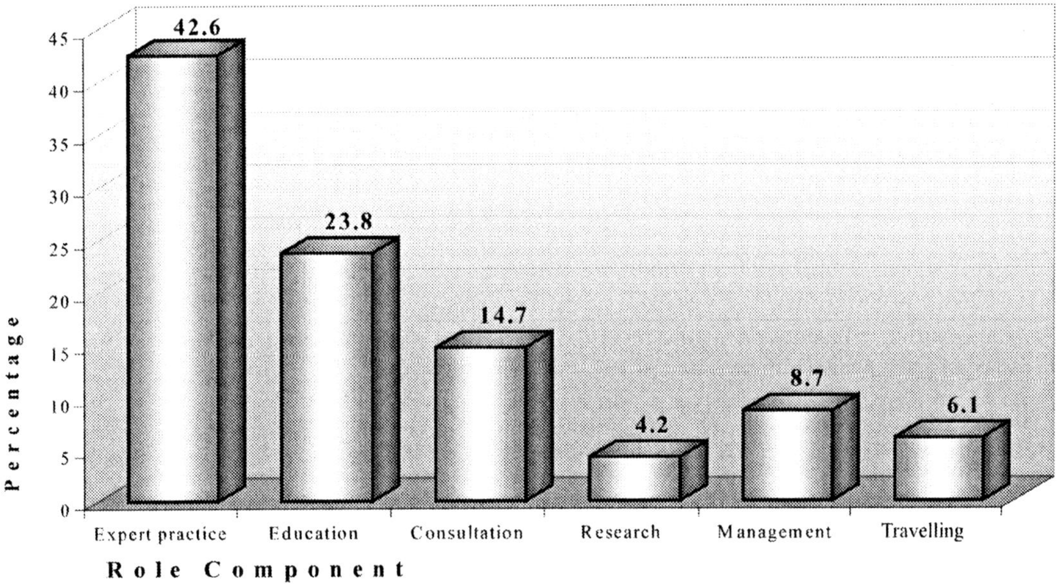

Figure 6.1 Percentage of total working time allotted to each role component (N=334)

A series of independent-samples t-tests were conducted to compare the percentage of time allotted to each role component for different groups of respondents. The mean percentages were compared for respondents working full-time as DSNs and those working part-time. There was a significant difference in the percentage of time allotted to expert practice, indicating that DSNs working full-time spent less time in this type of activity (Mean = 40.4%; SD = 15.4) than DSNs working part-time (Mean 48.5%, SD = 17.6; $t(332) = -4.09$, $p < 0.001$). This suggests that full-time DSNs have greater opportunity to develop other aspects of their role besides expert practice. Indeed, DSNs working full-time allotted more time to consultation (Mean = 15.7%; SD = 8.4) and research research (Mean = 4.6%; SD = 5.4) activities than DSNs working part-time (consultation activities—Mean = 12.1%, SD = 7.6; $t(332) = 3.56$, $p < 0.001$), (research activities—Mean = 3.1%, SD = 3.3; $t(332) = 2.38$, $p = 0.018$). Despite reaching statistical significance, the actual difference in mean scores between the groups was small. The effect size calculated using eta squared was 0.048 for expert practice, 0.037 for consultation, and 0.017 for research.

By conducting a one-way between-groups analysis of variance (ANOVA), a significant difference was found in the mean percentage of total working time that respondents spent in travelling ($F(2, 331) = 20.93$, $p < 0.001$). Post-hoc comparisons using the Tukey-HSD test suggested that DSNs working in hospital spent significantly less time in travelling (Mean = 3.9%; SD = 3.5) than DSNs working between hospital and community (Mean = 6.7%; SD = 4.4) and DSNs working in the community (Mean = 8.4%; SD = 5.3). The difference in the mean time percentages spent in travelling by DSNs working in each of the above three settings had a large effect size (eta squared = 0.112).

6.5 Discussion

6.5.1 Role components and activities

The results of this study confirmed the hypothesis derived from role theory that role performance is mutually interrelated with personal characteristics and skills, work setting and organisational factors, and positive phases of role development (see next chapter for details). Role performance, as explored in this study, consists of seven scales each measuring the following components of the DSN role: expert practice, education, consultation, research, management/leadership, collaboration/coordination, and innovation. These are now discussed.

6.5.1.1 Expert practice

Although the CNS involvement in direct care is considered a pivotal part of the role, the percentage of time allotted to its implementation has been reported as varied. Respondents in the present study reported that they allotted between 10% and 80% (Mean = 43%) of their total working time to expert practice activities. This study supports the findings reported in the literature that CNSs spent the majority of their time in expert practice. Several studies have shown that the majority spend approximately between 30% and 50% of their time in clinical practice (Malone, 1986; Robichaud and Hamric, 1986; Tarsitano *et al*, 1986; Walker, 1986). Scott (1999) reported that CNSs (N = 724) spent between 29% and 91% of the overall time required to undertake their role in clinical practice activities. Beecroft and Papenhausen (1985) (cited in Topham, 1987), in a survey of 262 CNSs, reported that 92% of the respondents spent more than 60% of their time in the clinician role.

Similar findings have also been reported by UK studies (Castledine *et al*, 1996; Johns, 1997). McGee and Castledine (1998), in their study, asked 280 chief nurses to list the work activities they expected CNSs to undertake. In a breakdown of activities related to clinical practice, 93% of the respondents expected CNSs to undertake specialised work, 87% direct care, 71% treating, 53% diagnosing, and 35% of them expected the CNS to undertake prescribing activities.

In this study, more than 90% of DSNs reported undertaking direct care either frequently or very frequently. Moreover, the majority of respondents undertook liaison and indirect care, and advanced specialised care either occasionally or frequently. Almost 60% of DSNs did not prescribe any diabetes-related medications. The majority of the remaining 40% commented that they were involved in this activity in the following forms: prescribing blood glucose strips, lancets and syringes; recommending treatment types and doses to medical colleagues; and/or filling in prescription forms for GPs and/or hospital doctors to sign. These forms of 'prescribing' have been previously reported by other authors (Brake, 1997; Padmore, 2000; Vick and Gardner, 2000). A recent study by James (2004) demonstrated the value of DSN prescribing in the acute setting, as it provided immediate support to people with diabetes and led to improved glycaemic control. However, although prescribing has been described as an important activity for the DSN, the issue of nurse prescribing unfortunately remains vague and has not been legalised (Brake, 1997; Padmore, 2000). The Department of Health (2003) recommended supplementary prescribing authority for DSNs, which is:

> *'A voluntary prescribing partnership between the independent prescriber and a supplementary prescriber, to implement an agreed patient-specific clinical management plan with the patient's agreement'.*

More than 80% of DSNs participated in interdisciplinary patient care conferences either occasionally, frequently or very frequently. Boyd *et al* (1991) found that the role of CNSs included coordinating, directing, and participating in the weekly multidisciplinary discharge planning patient care conferences. The purpose of the conferences was to coordinate the management of patient care during hospitalisation, and facilitate the implementation of the discharge plan by providing a link between patients and families, the hospital, and community resources. Furthermore, Young (1988) described the patient care conferences as a means for CNSs to use when entering into a new system or employment environment.

Varying allocations per role component may be related to the phase of role development (years of experience within the role). Baker (1987), in describing the developmental process of her role as a CNS, stated that the time she allotted to the clinician role component in the first two years ranged between 70–75% of the total time required for the role. Many studies have shown that the time CNSs spend in direct care decreases as they become more competent and confident within their role; more time is then allotted to other role components such as consultation and research (Cooper and Sparacino, 1990). Findings of the present study supported these assertions. A significant difference was found between DSNs employed for less than three years in their post and DSNs for more than fifteen years, indicating that the time allotted to expert practice activities decreased with long-term professional experience.

6.5.1.2 Education

A number of studies have reported that CNSs spent between 13% and 29% in the role of educator (Boyd *et al*, 1991; Naylor and Brooten, 1993; Robichaud and Hamric, 1986; Scott, 1997; Tarsitano *et al*, 1986). DSNs in the present study were closer to the higher end of the scale, allotting 24% of their total working time to education activities. This high percentage is probably due to the nature of diabetes as a chronic disease and the needs of patients, families, health staff and significant others for education. As DSNs are frequently assessing the clinical setting and changing and improving patient care, there is always a subject to teach. Most DSNs were involved in the education of patients and their families either frequently or very frequently.

In the study by Winocour *et al* (2002), including 351 consultant diabetologists across 238 NHS trusts/units in the UK, it was found that all DSNs working in these trusts were involved in diabetes education. Patient education took place predominantly (65%) as group sessions and on a one-to-one basis (34%). More than half of respondents reported that DSNs used written guidelines for the process of specialist input in patient education, but only 21% used formal written care plans.

DSNs also have a key role in the education of nursing staff and students, and the majority were involved in this activity either frequently or very frequently. The importance of this activity has also been demonstrated by previous studies (Farmer, 2000; Kyne-Grzebalski, 1997). It is interesting to note that more than 40% of DSNs provided education to medical staff and took part in the delivery of formal education frequently or very frequently. Similar findings were related to community or public information programmes. These findings are in contrast to those reported in a study involving 66 paediatric DSNs working across the UK, where the majority of respondents were not involved in this activity (Llahana *et al*, 2001a).

When new nurses enter the job market, they are considered novices in their ability to care for patients with various diagnoses across the life span. However, new graduate nurses require extensive and lengthy orientation, and their success is facilitated by the experienced, expert nurse who educates them in developing quality care for patients.

Scott (1997) asserts that CNSs are taught adult and paediatric learning theories in their graduate education which should prepare them to be more effective educators than nursing staff. CNSs incorporate these learning theories and strategies into educational programmes which ultimately yield successful learning environments that meet the needs of all healthcare professionals and students.

6.5.1.3 Consultation

According to the literature, CNSs spent approximately 8% to 18% of their total working time in the role of consultant (Boyd *et al*, 1991; Naylor and Brooten, 1993; Robichaud and Hamric, 1986; Scott, 1997). The CNS consultation has been described as 'a process in which an individual with recognised expertise is invited by another to assist in resolving a problem' (Hamric, 1983: p41). DSNs in this study allotted 15% of their total working time to consultation. An activity that most DSNs indicated they engaged in occasionally to frequently was collaboration with nurse managers to identify clinical activities to facilitate the professional growth of the nursing staff. Similar results were also reported by Scott (1997). This activity justifies specialist nurses remaining in collaborative relationships with nursing managers and not in subordinate relationships. Providing leadership in the development of policies and procedures, standards of care, protocols, and care pathways was another area highlighted in the DSNs' activities. According to Aitken *et al* (1990), CNSs have a strong influence on the development and implementation of hospital policies and programmes. They are frequently the initiators of policies, procedures, and protocols related to the areas of their expertise which have an impact on patient care services.

Scott (1997) reported that most CNSs in her study were involved in the facilitation of patient support groups either frequently or very frequently. The findings of the present study differ, as more than half of DSNs reported being either rarely or not at all involved in this activity. A number of authors have identified CNSs as leaders and facilitators of family support groups for critically ill patients, patients with significant heart disease and their partners. They are also recognised as leading and facilitating nurses' support groups (Ambutas, 1991; O'Keeffe and Gillis, 1988). In the present study, the majority of DSNs reported providing consultation for patients, their families and healthcare professionals either frequently or very frequently. According to Scott (1997), specialist nurses assist with these critical issues through role modelling, consulting, facilitating problem-solving and conflict resolution, and assuming advocacy roles for patients, families and health staff.

6.5.1.4 Research

DSNs in the present study spent the least percentage (4.2%) of their total working time in research activities. This percentage is lower than the range reported in the literature, which suggests that CNSs spent approximately 6% to 18% in the role of researcher (Boyd *et al*, 1991; Naylor and Brooten, 1993; Robichaud and Hamric, 1986; Scott, 1997). Although DSNs are in a prime position to be involved in research (Yallop, 1998), findings of the present and other relevant studies (Humphris *et al*, 1999; Scott, 1999) do not support this. However, as McGee and Castledine (1999) reported, more than 60% of chief nurses expected CNSs to undertake research activities. Reasons for DSNs' low involvement in research were not identified, as this was not an objective of this study. However, workload pressures, time and resource limitations and lack of research knowledge were some of the basic barriers reported by a previous study which involved 299 DSNs (Humphris *et al*, 1999).

Collins (1992) noted that the reason for the research role remaining a low priority is because CNSs are not academically prepared at the Master's level to conduct research, and therefore, shy away from research and may even fear it. In the present study, only 22% of DSNs held a Master's degree. Scott (1997) stated that another reason could be that research is a time-intensive endeavour, and the multifaceted nature of the CNS practice means that practitioners might not have the time to implement the researcher role as fully as they implement the other role components.

Despite this, DSNs in this study were heavily engaged in disseminating research findings to the nursing staff, collaborating with other health professionals in research, and using the research process for product evaluations. These research activities were also supported by Collins (1992) and Aikin *et al* (1993). More than 56% of DSNs in this study identified nursing care problems and developed questions for systematic study. This activity was supported by several authors as a role of the CNS. They contend that, through clinical expertise and knowledge of research methodology, the CNS can identify clinical problems that can be addressed through research utilisation (Beaudry *et al*, 1996; Humphris *et al*, 1999; Ryan-Merritt *et al*, 1988; Scott, 1997).

With advanced preparation at Master's level, and the focus on research conduct and utilisation in their graduate programmes, CNSs are the ideal resources, in comparison with general nurses, to facilitate the incorporation of research findings into the practice area, thereby assisting in the linkage between clinical practice and nursing research. It has been acknowledged that CNSs utilise research and change practice on the basis of research findings (Collins, 1992; Stetler and DiMaggio, 1991; Utz and Gleit, 1995).

6.5.1.5 Management/leadership

According to the literature, approximately 6% to 25% of the CNS's time is spent in the role of administrator (Boyd *et al*, 1991; Naylor and Brooten, 1993; Robichaud and Hamric, 1986; Scott, 1997). DSNs in the present study allotted 8.4% of their total working time to management and leadership activities. This finding does not support Sparacino (1990), who stated that CNSs utilised the administrator role the least.

As in research, the majority of DSNs responded to the question regarding the frequency with which they undertook management activities with 'Not at all', 'Rarely' or 'Occasionally'. An exception was the activity 'Participate in identifying gaps in the diabetes care services', which almost 50% of DSNs reported undertaking either frequently or very frequently. However, this role component, as reported by McGee and Castledine (1999), was greatly valued by the nursing administration; more than 70% of chief nurses in their study expected CNSs to be involved in administrative activities. The DSNs in this study identified that the management and leadership activity in which they engaged frequently was the identification of gaps in diabetes care services. A number of DSNs in this study reported that they had undertaken a large amount of administrative responsibilities, which inhibited the performance of their other role components. Given these findings, the activities of a DSN/nurse manager could potentially lean more heavily towards managerial responsibilities rather than towards clinical responsibilities.

6.5.1.6 Collaboration/coordination and innovation

As noted in previous chapters, respondents were not asked to estimate the percentages of their total work time that they spent in collaboration and innovation, as these activities often overlap with the five components described above. Mixed responses were given by DSNs regarding the frequency with which they undertook each of the activities that constitute the components of collaboration and innovation. However, the majority reported undertaking these role components either frequently or very frequently.

Hamric (1989) views collaboration and innovation as competencies of the CNS rather than distinct role components, because the CNS utilises these in all the other role components. However, for the purposes of their investigation, these competencies have been treated as role components in the present study. Collaboration between different care settings is a vital aspect of the DSN role because of the chronic nature of diabetes, and is crucial to providing continuous and comprehensive care for patients and their families. The DSN has a key role in its facilitation. Hamric (1989) maintains that collaboration requires skill in communication and in maintaining effective interpersonal relationships. The importance of communication and interpersonal skills in the DSN practice was highlighted and discussed earlier in this chapter. Central to the position of the CNS is the role of change agent, as their purpose is to change and improve aspects of their practice relating to patient care. Fenton (1985) reported that the CNS is the most creative and appropriate professional in developing ways to institute change in an organisation that resists change.

6.6 Summary

The DSN role performance was explored in this chapter. The instrument used for the data collection was based on the CNS literature and specifically modified to fit the DSN role. The exploratory factor analysis revealed that this instrument presents a reliable measurement of the DSN role performance. Respondents reported being highly involved in expert practice, education and consultation. However, they spent the least of their time in research and management activities.

It is important to stress that, although all the role components are essential, the time allotted to each depends on the DSN job description and work setting. It also depends on the expectations imposed on DSNs by the organisation, administration, peers, staff nurses and other health professionals, as well as the immediate needs of patients and their families. Moreover, as pointed out earlier, it is unrealistic to expect DSNs to perform all components from the start of their career or simultaneously at any stage of their role development. The temptation to be everywhere at once and all things to all people may be strong, particularly for the novice CNS. However, as Cameron (1994) pointed out, giving in to this urge could render the CNS a physical wreck at best, and a dabbler at worst. Additionally, as different activities combining each of the role components are interconnected and often overlap, they are equally important and, thus, difficult to separate into discrete components.

The next chapter brings together all the CNS role concepts explored in previous chapters and examines the associations among them. A multiple regression model is used to test the theoretical framework underpinning this study to develop a valid framework for the DSN role.

7

A valid theoretical framework for the role of the diabetes specialist nurse and implications and recommendations for nursing practice

7.1 Introduction

The role of the clinical nurse specialist (CNS) was explored in the previous chapters of this book guided by a theoretical framework derived from role theory. The evolution and definition of the CNS role in the USA and the UK were presented in the first chapter, while the second chapter explored the relevance of role theory to the CNS role. The following four concepts constituting the theoretical framework of the CNS role derived from role theory were examined in a UK-nationwide study involving 334 diabetes specialist nurses (DSN) and discussed in *Chapters 3* to *6*:

1. Personal characteristics and skills
2. Work setting and organisational factors
3. Role development (positive phases, negative phases)
4. Role performance

The associations between the dimensions of these concepts (parameters) are explored in this chapter. In addition, the following hypotheses about the DSN role in the UK were made in *Chapter 2*, examining the relevance of role theory to clinical specialist nursing:

- The DSN role performance is influenced by their personal characteristics and skills, by work setting and organisational factors related to their role, and by the process of their role development
- The parameters related to the DSN role, role performance, personal characteristics and skills, work setting and organisational factors, and role development, are mutually interrelated.

These hypotheses are tested in the first part of this chapter in relation to the DSN role and a valid theoretical framework is developed to explain this role.

Findings and the strengths and limitation of this study are discussed in the second part of the chapter. The implications of this study for nursing practice and recommendations for administration, education and future research are made in the final part.

This chapter brings together all the CNS role concepts explored in this book to test and develop a valid theoretical framework. Therefore, the reader is strongly advised to read the previous chapters in order to understand the associations between the concepts presented in this chapter, the value of the theoretical framework and the implications of this study for nursing practice. A detailed description of each concept goes beyond the scope of this chapter.

7.2 Associations between different parameters of the study

One of the objectives of this study was to explore the associations between the different CNS role concepts as applied to the diabetes speciality. The relationship between the dimensions of the Personal Characteristics and Skills Scale and those of the Work Setting Factors Scale was investigated using Pearson's product-moment correlation test. The results presented in *Table 7.1* show a number of low positive correlations at the $p < 0.01$ level of significance between the factors constituting the above scales.

All three factors of personal characteristics and skills correlated significantly with collaborative working. This enhances the importance of the acquisition of these characteristics by the DSN in the achievement of optimum working relationships with other health professionals. A high correlation was found between organisational issues and role expectations ($r = 0.391$; $p < 0.001$), suggesting that respondents were more able to effect change when their expectations were compatible with those of the employing organisation.

Table 7.1 Examination of the relationships between factors constituting the scales of personal characteristics and skills and work setting factors using Pearson's correlation coefficient r test (N=334)

Factor		Work Setting Factors Factor 1: Collaborative Working	Work Setting Factors Factor 2: Role expectations	Work Setting Factors Factor 3: Resources
Personal Characteristics Factor 1: Competence within Role	Pearson r	*.220****	*.126**	*.041*
	Sig. p	*.000*	*.021*	*.455*
Personal Characteristics Factor 2: Organisational Issues	Pearson r	*.185***	*.391****	*.150***
	Sig. p	*.001*	*.000*	*.006*
Personal Characteristics Factor 3: Personal Attributes	Pearson r	*.176***	*.045*	*.067*
	Sig. p	*.001*	*.412*	*.224*

*Correlation is significant at the 0.05 level (2-tailed)
**Correlation is significant at the 0.01 level (2-tailed)
***Correlation is significant at the 0.001 level (2-tailed)

The relationships between the seven components constituting role performance and the factors combined within the Personal Characteristics and Skills Scale and the Work Setting Factors Scale were also explored using Pearson's correlation test (*Table 7.2*). Most role components correlated at the $p < 0.001$ level of significance with factors of the Personal Characteristics and Skills Scale. Findings indicate that respondents who rated more highly their personal characteristics related to the DSN role undertook the activities included in their role at a higher frequency. More specifically, a large number of moderate correlations ($p < 0.01$) was found between role components and respondents' competence within role and personal attributes. However, a small number of correlations at a lower level of significance ($p < 0.05$) was found between work setting factors and the different role components. This indicates that respondents associated the optimal performance of their role more closely with their personal characteristics than with factors derived from their work setting.

Pearson's correlation test was also used to explore the relationships between role development and the dimensions of the following parameters examined in this study: personal characteristics and skills, work setting and organisational factors, and role performance. As reported in *Chapter 5*, the developmental phases were categorised in two distinct (non-correlated) groups, positive phases and negative phases. For this reason, any further statistical analysis exploring the association of role development with other parameters examined in this study considered the above two groups of developmental phases separately.

Table 7.2 Examination of the relationships between components constituting role performance and factors constituting the scales of personal characteristics and skills and work setting factors using Pearson's correlation coefficient r test (N=334)

Factor *Role Component*		Expert Practice	Education	Consult-ation	Research	Manage-ment	Collabor-ation	Innovation
Personal Characteristics Factor 1: Competence within Role	Pearson r Sig. p	.303*** .000	.249*** .000	.442*** .000	.392*** .000	.376*** .000	.189** .001	.368*** .000
Personal Characteristics Factor 2: Organisational Issues	Pearson r Sig. p	.059 .282	.033 .545	.169** .002	.222*** .000	.233*** .000	.096 .080	.204*** .000
Personal Characteristics Factor 3: Personal Attributes	Pearson r Sig. p	.351*** .000	.285*** .000	.340*** .000	.355*** .000	.225*** .000	.328*** .000	.305*** .000
Work Setting Factors Factor 1: Collaborative Working	Pearson r Sig. p	.113* .039	.052 .343	.098 .072	.095 .083	.160** .003	.041 .458	.066 .229
Work Setting Factors Factor 2: Role expectations	Pearson r Sig. p	.138* .011	.128* .019	.071 .198	.052 .347	.042 .445	.038 .490	.033 .544
Work Setting Factors Factor 3: Resources	Pearson r Sig. p	.121* .027	.076 .165	.048 .384	.043 .433	.113* .039	.053 .330	.011 .842

As seen in *Table 7.3,* the experience of positive phases by respondents was closely associated with the different parameters related to the DSN role. A high positive correlation at the $p < 0.001$ level of significance was found between positive phases and most role components indicating that DSNs who reported experience of the integration and implementation phases (combined within this group) were involved in different role activities at a higher frequency.

Table 7.3 Examination of the relationships between role development and personal characteristics and skills, work setting factors, and role performance using Pearson's correlation coefficient r test (N=334)

Scale	*Correlation Test*	**Role Development** Positive phases	**Role Development** Negative phases
Personal Characteristics Factor 1: Competence within Role	Pearson r Sig. p	*.287**** *.000*	*.072* *.191*
Personal Characteristics Factor 2: Organisational Issues	Pearson r Sig. p	*.192**** *.000*	*-.198**** *.000*
Personal Characteristics Factor 3: Personal Attributes	Pearson r Sig. p	*.215**** *.000*	*.082* *.137*
Work Setting Factors Factor 1: Collaborative Working	Pearson r Sig. p	*.113** *.039*	*-.180*** *.001*
Work Setting Factors Factor 2: Role expectations	Pearson r Sig. p	*.117** *.032*	*-.456**** *.000*
Work Setting Factors Factor 3: Resources	Pearson r Sig. p	*.105* *.055*	*-.160*** *.003*
Role Component Expert Practice	Pearson r Sig. p	*.219**** *.000*	*.147*** *.007*
Role Component Education	Pearson r Sig. p	*.233**** *.000*	*.104* *.057*
Role Component Consultation	Pearson r Sig. p	*.399**** *.000*	*.142** *.010*
Role Component Research	Pearson r Sig. p	*.350**** *.000*	*.003* *.957*
Role Component Management/leadership	Pearson r Sig. p	*.354**** *.000*	*.040* *.463*
Role Component Collaboration/coordination	Pearson r Sig. p	*.208**** *.000*	*.077* *.159*
Role Component Innovation	Pearson r Sig. p	*.379**** *.000*	*.017* *.761*

* Correlation is significant at the 0.05 level (2-tailed).
** Correlation is significant at the 0.01 level (2-tailed).
*** Correlation is significant at the 0.001 level (2-tailed).

On the other hand, negative correlations at the $p < 0.001$ level of significance were reported between work setting factors and negative phases. More specifically, a high correlation was found between the latter and role expectations ($r = -0.456$, $p < 0.001$), indicating that incongruent expectations were closely associated with the experience of anxiety and role strain by respondents. However, the experience of negative phases did not correlate with respondents' performance of the different role components. This suggests that negative experiences of role development act as barriers to CNS's adequate role performance.

7.3 Testing the theoretical framework underpinning the study of the DSN role

In *Chapter 2,* which described the theoretical framework underpinning the present study, it was asserted that all the parameters constituting this framework reciprocally influence one another. However, as described in previous chapters, only the following parameters of this framework were explored in the present study: personal characteristics and skills, work setting and organisational factors influencing role performance, role performance, and role development (positive and negative phases).

The ultimate objective of the present study was to test the hypotheses derived from the role theory CNS theoretical framework of the above parameters when exploring DSN role influence and/or their potential to predict each other. Standard multiple regression was used to examine the prediction of each of the above parameters by other parameters involved in this study.

Prior to conducting multiple regression analysis, the relationships between the above parameters were examined using Pearson's correlation test. The results are presented in *Table 7.4*, where it can be seen that most parameters in this study correlated significantly with each other. The highest correlation was found between personal characteristics and role performance. A moderate negative correlation was found between work setting factors and negative phases. This suggests that respondents related the negative experiences of their role development to the limited support from their work setting in the facilitation of their role performance.

Table 7.4 Examination of the relationships between the parameters related to the DSN role using Pearson's correlation coefficient r test (N = 334)

Study Parameter		Positive Phases	Negative Phases	Personal Characteristics	Work Setting Factors	Role Components
Role Development Positive Phases	Pearson r Sig. p	1.000				
Role Development Negative Phases	Pearson r Sig. p	.043 .437	1.000			
Personal Characteristics & Skills	Pearson r Sig. p	.324*** .000	-.052 .344	1.000		
Work Setting Factors	Pearson r Sig. p	.149** .006	-.397*** .000	.351*** .000	1.000	
Role Performance Role Components	Pearson r Sig. p	.432*** .000	.118* .031	.178*** .000	.017 .752	1.000

* Correlation is significant at the 0.05 level (2-tailed).
** Correlation is significant at the 0.01 level (2-tailed).
*** Correlation is significant at the 0.001 level (2-tailed).

Pearson's correlation coefficient indicated the strength and direction of the relationships between the study parameters, but did not indicate causality. That is, for two correlated parameters, it was not possible to indicate which one predicted the other. This was achieved in the present study through multiple regression analysis. Moreover, Pearson's correlation test takes into consideration the relationship between only two variables. Hence, an additional advantage of multiple regression in relation to this study was the potential to evaluate the prediction of a particular parameter from a set of others.

Five analyses were conducted in order to test how well the following parameters included in the theoretical framework underpinning the present study predicted (influenced) each other:

1. Role performance (role components);
2. Personal characteristics and skills ;
3. Work setting and organisational factors;
4. Role development (positive developmental phases); and
5. Role development (negative developmental phases).

7.3.1 Prediction of role performance

Two questions were answered in this section:

a) How well is role performance predicted by the other four parameters explored in the present study? and

b) Which of the four parameters is the best predictor for role performance?

The above five parameters were put into a standard multiple regression analysis with role performance as the dependent variable. The results presented in *Table 7.5* show a high correlation ($r = 0.590$; $p < 0.001$) between the four predictors combined and the dependent parameter (role performance). The value of r square (0.348) indicates that the four predictor parameters (personal characteristics and skills, work setting and organisational factors, positive phases, negative phases) explain 34.8% of the variance in role performance.

Table 7.5 Multiple regression analysis exploring the prediction of role performance of the DSN by other parameters involved in the study (N = 334)

Dependent Variable	Role Performance (Role Components)		
Predictors	Beta (β)	t-test (t)	Significance (p)
Personal Characteristics and Skills	.435	8.732	.000
Work Setting and Organisational Factors	.156	2.992	.003
Role Development (Positive Phases)	.312	6.596	.000
Role Development (Negative Phases)	.065	1.332	.184
Model Summary: r = .590; r square = .348; adjusted r square = .340; F(4, 329) = 43.87, p < .001			

The adjusted r square value of 0.340 suggests that the above predictors account for 34% of the variance in role performance when results are applied to the population from which the study sample was drawn. As the difference between the values of r square and adjusted r square is minimal, it can be concluded that the findings of this regression model can be generalised very well to the overall population of DSNs. This model is highly significant ($p < 0.001$), and the large value of $F = 43.87$ (greater than 1) suggests that this result is very unlikely to have happened by chance.

With regard to question b, personal characteristics and skills made the strongest statistically significant unique contribution to predicting role performance ($\beta = 0.435$; $p < 0.001$), when the effects of all other predictor parameters were held constant. Positive phases of role development and work setting factors also made a significant contribution to predicting role performance. All three predictors had a positive influence on the dependent parameter (positive β values). This means that the more highly respondents rated these predictor parameters, the more frequently they were involved in activities constituting role performance. In contrast, negative phases of role development did not add to the ability to predict role performance, since the level of significance p is greater than 0.05. This indicates that the experience of negative feelings by respondents during the process of their role development did not have an impact on the performance of their role.

7.3.2 Prediction of personal characteristics and skills

A multiple regression analysis with personal characteristics and skills as the dependent variable was used to answer the following two questions:

a) How well are personal characteristics and skills related to the DSN role by the other four parameters explored in the present study? and

b) Which of the four parameters is the best predictor for personal characteristics and skills?

The results presented in *Table 7.6* show a high correlation ($r = 0.594$; $p < 0.001$) between the four predictors combined and the dependent variable (personal characteristics and skills). The regression model represented by the four predictor-parameters in this section explained 35.3% of the variance in personal characteristics and skills (r square = 0.353). The estimate of the explained variance in the dependent variable by this model for the population from which the sample was drawn was 34.5% (adjusted r square = 0.345). The minimal difference between the values of r square and adjusted r square indicates that these findings can be generalised very well to the overall population of DSNs. In addition, this model presented a high level of significance ($F = 44.78$; $p < 0.001$), which indicates that it is very unlikely that this result has been reached by chance.

Table 7.6 Multiple regression analysis exploring the prediction of personal characteristics and skills of the DSN by other parameters examined in this study (N = 334)

Dependent Variable	Personal Characteristics and Skills		
Predictors	Beta (β)	t-test (t)	Significance (p)
Work Setting and Organisational Factors	.342	6.964	.000
Role Development (Positive Phases)	.085	1.694	.091
Role Development (Negative Phases)	.029	.601	.548
Role Performance (Role Components)	.432	8.732	.000

Model Summary:
r = .594; r square = .353; adjusted r square = .345; F(4, 329) = 44.78, p < .001

Role performance made the strongest significant unique contribution in the prediction of personal characteristics and skills in this model ($\beta = 0.432$; $p < 0.001$), when the effect of the other three predictors remained constant. A similar result was reported in the previous section, where it was seen that personal characteristics and skills made the strongest contribution to predicting role performance. This suggests a mutual influence between these two parameters, i.e. the more frequently DSNs undertook activities constituting their role performance, the higher they rated their personal characteristics and skills, and vice versa.

Work setting factors also had a significant influence on the prediction of personal characteristics and skills ($\beta = 0.342$; $p < 0.001$). The remaining two predictors included in role development, however, did not add to the ability to predict the dependent variable in this model ($p > 0.05$). This indicates that respondents' personal characteristics and skills were not influenced by the experience of positive or negative phases.

7.3.3 Prediction of work setting and organisational factors

Two questions were answered in this section:

a) How well is the dependent parameter work setting and organisational factors predicted by the other four parameters involved in this study? and

b) Which of the four parameters is the best predictor for work setting factors?

The results obtained from standard multiple regression analysis (*Table 7.7*) revealed a high correlation between the four predictor parameters combined and work setting factors ($r = 0.538$; $p < 0.001$). The value of r square = 0.290 in this regression model shows that 29% of the variance in the dependent variable (work setting factors) is accounted for by the predictors. On the basis of the adjusted r square value of 0.281, it can be concluded that this model can be generalised very well to the overall population of DSNs. That is, predictor parameters account for 28.1% of the variance in work setting factors when results are applied to the target population. This model presents a high level of significance ($F = 33.58$; $p < 0.001$).

Table 7.7 Multiple regression analysis exploring the prediction of work setting factors related to the DSN role by other parameters involved in the study (N = 334)

Dependent Variable	Work setting and organisational factors		
Predictors	Beta (β)	t-test (t)	Significance (p)
Personal Characteristics and Skills	*.375*	*6.964*	*.000*
Role Development (Positive Phases)	*.117*	*2.237*	*.026*
Role Development (Negative Phases)	*-.362*	*-7.686*	*.000*
Role Performance (Role Components)	*.170*	*2.992*	*.003*
Model Summary: r = .538; r square = .290; adjusted r square = .281; F(4, 329) = 33.58, p < .001			

All the predictor parameters in this model made a significant contribution to predicting work setting factors, with the strongest recorded for personal characteristics and skills ($\beta = 0.375$; $p < 0.001$). Negative phases of role development had a negative significant influence on the prediction of work setting factors ($\beta = -0.362$; $p < 0.001$), indicating that respondents associated closely the experience of these phases with the limited support from their working environment.

7.3.4 Prediction of role development (positive phases)

Two questions were answered in this section after running a standard multiple regression analysis with positive phases of role development as the dependent variable (parameter):

a) How well is role development (positive phases) predicted by the other four parameters involved in the present study? and

b) Which of the four parameters is the best predictor for positive phases?

The results of this analysis (*Table 7.8*) revealed a moderate correlation ($r = 0.465$; $p < 0.001$) between the four predictor parameters combined and positive phases of role development (dependent parameter). The predictor parameters in this regression model accounted for 21.7% (r square = 0.217) of the variance in positive phases. Moreover, generalisation of findings is possible, as this model can explain 20.7% of the variance in the dependent parameter when applied to the overall population of DSNs (adjusted r square = 0.207). The regression model in this section reached a high level of statistical significance ($F = 22.73$; $p < 0.001$).

Table 7.8 Multiple regression analysis exploring the prediction of the positive role development of the DSN by other parameters included in this study (N = 334)

Dependent variable	Role development (positive phases)		
Predictors	Beta (β)	t-test (t)	Significance (p)
Personal characteristics and skills	.102	1.694	.091
Work setting and organisational factors	.129	2.237	.026
Role development (negative phases)	.055	1.021	.308
Role performance (role components)	.375	6.596	.000
Model summary: r = .465; r square = .217; adjusted r square = .207; F(4, 329) = 22.73, p < .001			

The strongest unique significant contribution in the prediction of positive phases in this model was made by role performance (β = 0.375; p < 0.001). This suggests that respondents who undertook role activities at a higher frequency than other respondents reported a greater extent of experience of implementation and integration phases. Work setting factors also had a significant impact on the prediction of positive phases, although at a lower level of significance than role performance (β = 129; p = 0.026). On the other hand, personal characteristics and skills, as well as negative phases, did not make a significant contribution in the prediction of positive phases. This finding was, in fact, expected for negative phases because, as reported earlier, they did not correlate with positive phases.

7.3.5 Prediction of negative phases of role development

The final standard multiple regression analysis in this section, with negative phases of role development as the dependent variable, answered the following two questions:

a) How well is role performance (negative phases) predicted by the other four parameters involved in the present study? and

b) Which of the four parameters is the best predictor for negative phases?

As presented in *Table 7.9*, a moderate correlation (r = 0.421; p < 0.001) was found between the four predictor parameters combined and the negative phases of role development (dependent parameter). However, only 17.7% of the total variance in negative phases was explained by the predictor parameters in this regression model (r square = 0.177). An inspection of the beta values revealed that work setting factors was the only parameter in this model that made a unique significant contribution to predicting negative phases (β = -0.420; p < 0.001). The negative value suggests a negative relationship between the two parameters. That is, respondents who had limited or no support from their work setting in the facilitation of their role reported a greater extent of negative phases experience.

Table 7.9 Multiple regression analysis exploring the prediction of the negative role development of the DSN by other parameters included in this study (N = 334)

Dependent variable	Role development (negative phases)		
Predictors	Beta (β)	t-test (t)	Significance (p)
Personal characteristics and skills	*.037*	*.601*	*.548*
Work setting and organisational factors	*-.420*	*-7.686*	*.000*
Role development (positive phases)	*.058*	*1.021*	*.308*
Role performance (role components)	*.082*	*1.332*	*.184*
Model summary: r = .421; r square =.177; adjusted r square = .167; $F(4, 329) = 17.68$, $p < .001$			

The regression model in this section reached a high level of statistical significance ($F = 17.68$; $p < 0.001$), indicating that this result did not happen by chance. Moreover, the small difference between the values of the r square (0.177) and the adjusted r square (0.167) allows for generalisation of findings. This model has the ability to explain 16.7% of the total variance in negative phases when applied to the overall population of DSNs.

7.4. A valid theoretical framework for the DSN role

This chapter examined the relationships between the dimensions of the DSN role-related parameters explored in the present study. A close association was found between most dimensions. In addition, the hypothesis derived from the theoretical framework underpinning the study (*Chapter 2*) suggesting mutual interrelationships between the following role parameters was challenged:

1. Personal characteristics and skills;
2. Work setting and organisational factors;
3. Role development (positive phases, negative phases); and
4. Role performance.

The theoretical framework derived from the role theory field was modified based on the results of this study to explain the role of the DSN in the UK (*Figure 7.1*).

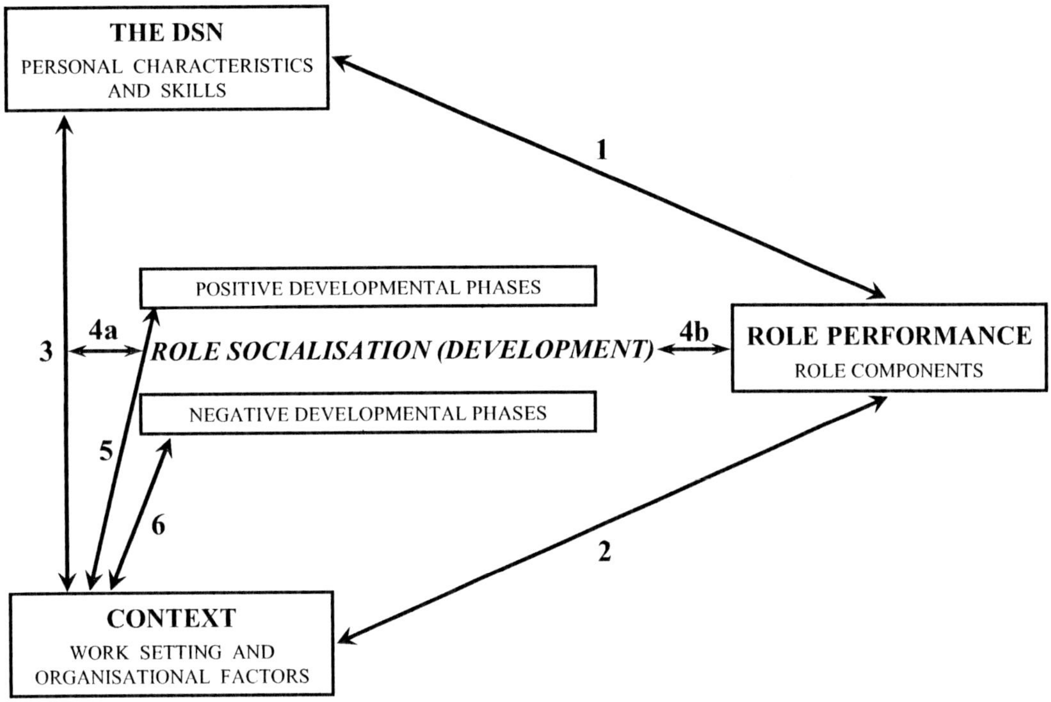

Figure 7.1 The theoretical framework underpinning the present study modified on the basis of results obtained from Stage 1 of the study

The following results were obtained with respect to the five parameters relating to the DSN role as they are combined within the above framework:

1. Role performance (role components) is influenced by the following parameters (presented in descending order based on the level of significance of their prediction):
   - Personal characteristics and skills of the DSN (arrow 1)
   - Positive phases of role development (arrow 4)
   - Work setting and organisational factors related to the DSN role (arrow 2)
2. Personal characteristics and skills are influenced by the following parameters:
   - Role performance (role components) of the DSN (arrow 1)
   - Work setting and organisational factors related to the DSN role (arrow 3)
3. Work setting and organisational factors are influenced by the following parameters:
   - Personal characteristics and skills of the DSN (arrow 3)
   - Negative phases of role development (arrow 6)
   - Role performance (role components) of the DSN (arrow 2)
   - Positive phases of role development (arrow 5)

4. Role development (positive developmental phases) of the DSN is influenced by the following parameters:
   - Role performance (role components) of the DSN (arrow 4)
   - Work setting and organisational factors related to the DSN role (arrow 5)
5. Role development (negative developmental phases) of the DSN is influenced by the following parameter:
   - Work setting and organisational factors related to the DSN role (arrow 6)

7.5 Discussion

Although the findings of this study support the assertion by Watkinson (1997) that a combination of clinical experience, advanced education and high level of personal characteristics and skills constitute an expert DSN, this is not always enough. The present study showed that for an expert DSN to be able to maximise his or her role-related personal attributes and competencies, appropriate support must be provided by other parties within the work setting, such as administration, peers and health professionals. Material support is also vital. These findings were confirmed by comments from DSNs. Factors deriving from the work setting were cited as the main reasons for the varied feelings of DSNs during their role development. These factors had either a positive or negative impact on their personal values, attitudes and motives regarding the DSN role; that is, they experienced either job satisfaction or role strain.

The association between the personal characteristics of CNSs and factors derived from their work settings has been very little explored (Bousfield, 1997; Hamric and Taylor, 1989; McFadden and Miller, 1994). However, the reciprocal influence between individuals' personal values, characteristics and competencies and their social environments was highlighted by role theorists as early as the 1930s. Linton (1936) maintained that individuals and their behaviours are both shaped by their social environment, but they can also change and mould their environment under favourable conditions. Many DSNs in this study stated that their personal characteristics, such as tolerance, patience and determination, had helped them to avoid any negative impact on their personality of the different constraints deriving from the work setting. As discussed in *Chapter 5*, exploring the role development process, these constraints resulted in incongruence between the role expectations imposed on DSNs and their own perception of role.

Role theorists also posit that a reciprocal influence exists between individuals' personal characteristics and their role socialisation (development). Individuals learn to perform their roles adequately through socialisation, which, in turn, depends to a great extent on the role-learning abilities and the intelligence level of each individual (Biddle, 1979; Hurley-Wilson, 1988). However, the results of the present study rejected the hypothesis that there is a mutual relationship between role-related skills and personal attributes of DSNs and the process of role socialisation.

This is shown by the multiple regression analysis used to test the theoretical framework of the CNS role, which revealed that personal characteristics and skills were not influenced by role development (positive phases and negative phases) and vice versa. Although most dimensions of the personal characteristics scale correlated significantly with the developmental phases, it is important to stress that this does not indicate causality between the parameters.

It is worth noting that the association between the above parameters has not been previously explored in the nursing literature. Further investigation is needed to test the hypothesis that DSN personality and role-related skills, and the process of their role socialisation, are mutually dependent. In the present study, the exploration of the role development process was considered on the basis of DSNs' experiences within role and their feelings arising from this process. Other nurse researchers have also explored the nurse role development on the basis of skill acquisition (Baker, 1987; Benner, 2001; Holt, 1987). Therefore, any generalisations of findings of the present study refer exclusively to the experiences and feelings of CNSs during the process of their role development.

Findings of the present study supported the assertion made by role theorists that individuals' role performance is shaped by contextual factors, such as material resources, organisational issues and interpersonal relationships with significant others (Biddle, 1979; Katz and Kahn, 1978). Conway (1988b) contends that it is important for health professionals to understand the structure and nature of healthcare organisations in order to cope adequately with problems that may arise in relation to their role performance. The reciprocal influence between individuals' personal characteristics and their social environments has also been explored in the role theory field. Although the nursing literature relating to this topic is limited, findings of this study affirmed the above association. In fact, personal characteristics and skills were found to be the best predictor for work setting and organisational factors, compared to other role-related parameters tested in this study.

Role theorists support that the process of role socialisation is determined by a third-party standpoint, indicating the performance expected of the role occupant. This third party may be a person, or a group of people, or may be depersonalised into a norm or expectation (Turner, 1966). This is in accordance with the findings of the present study, which suggest that a reciprocal influence exists between work setting and organisational factors and the role development process, i.e. experience of developmental phases by DSNs. This influence presented a higher level of significance in relation to negative phases ($\beta = -0.362$; $p < 0.001$) than to positive phases ($\beta = 0.117$; $p = 0.026$).

This indicates that, although work setting factors are responsible for the experience of both the negative and positive phases, their prediction is more powerfully related to the negative phases. That is to say, CNSs are more prone to experiencing feelings such as anxiety and frustration in the presence of constraints and/or conflicts arising from their work setting. These findings were illustrated in the comments made by DSNs regarding the process of their role development. As discussed in *Chapter 5*, they identified factors arising from their work setting as major determinants for the experience of these negative developmental phases. Similar findings were reported by Hamric and Taylor (1989).

7.6 Strengths and limitations of the study exploring the DSN role

7.6.1 The value and limitations of using a theoretical framework

The theoretical framework underpinning this study was derived from the role theory field. From the discussion in *Chapter 2* exploring the elements of this framework, it is maintained that research lacking in theoretical soundness is of little practical use in the development of a professional and scientific knowledge base. Moody (1990: p239) maintained that the contribution of theory-isolated research to knowledge is limited and '...may result in isolated fact collecting and never contribute to theoretical progress in an area.'

The concept of the CNS role, including that of the DSN, is very broad and much has been written about its key elements and components. Until the present study, no theory has been generated to describe and explain the relationships between the parameters that constitute this role. The existence of this gap in the nursing literature made the generation of a theoretical framework a necessity in order to accomplish the goal of this study and provide an in-depth exploration of the DSN role. The use of concepts derived from the role theory field to construct this framework was the most appropriate, as role theory is related to the study of human behaviour (Biddle, 1979).

However, while the theoretical framework guided this study, it is acknowledged that there are problems inherent in this, and its use was not without limitations. It can, therefore, be argued that, while the theoretical framework used appears to 'fit' the DSN role, it may not be the only one to do so. Sometimes, there may be more than one theory to explain the same phenomenon (Parahoo, 1997), which may not necessarily be better or worse. A clear description of the rationale for adopting concepts from role theory to guide this study is given in *Chapter 2*.

This theoretical framework guided the exploration of human behaviour and enactment in a role (Biddle, 1979) and, thus, it cannot be totally devoid of human perspective which is, inevitably, changeable. Moreover, it is evident that the CNS role is rapidly progressing, and its flexible nature means that its definition changes according to prevailing circumstances. Therefore, although in the present study the use of this framework was significant, there is a possibility that this may not be the case when tested with a different CNS population and context or after ten years with the same population. The strength of the theoretical framework in this study is that it provided a structured and theoretically underpinned mapping of the examined elements constituting the DSN role.

The theoretical framework derived from role theory relevant to the exploration of the DSN role comprised the following six mutually interrelated concepts:

- Personal characteristics of the DSN
- Context for role performance
- Role socialisation (development)
- Role performance
- Role expectations
- Role stress and role strain.

However, due to time and financial constraints, only the first four concepts and their relations to each other were explored. This presented a limitation to this study and it cannot be asserted that the patterns of their interrelations would remain unchangeable under the impact of role expectations and role stress and role strain.

Despite the limitations, this theoretical framework provided tangible guidance and consistency throughout this study. The present study provided the nursing literature with an empirically tested, theoretical framework that can be used in further exploration of the CNS role. The results of this study suggested that findings could be generalised, and, thus, the framework can also be utilised in the study of other CNS roles. Nevertheless, this theoretical framework clearly requires further intensive and rigorous testing before its components can be wholly adopted as the basis for CNS practice.

7.6.2 Strengths and limitations of the study design and instrument

This was the first nation-wide study to explore the role performance and development of the DSN in the UK and the factors influencing them. Findings suggested that the DSN role has been clearly established in the UK although there are still many areas which need to be enhanced. In addition, it was found that the role development and implementation of the DSN role present close similarities to those of the CNS as documented in the literature. The strength of this study is that it provided a comprehensive exploration of the parameters related to the DSN role and the interrelations between them.

The large study sample (653 DSNs), the statistically significant response rate (over 50%), and the strength of the data analysis (high internal consistency of scales within the study instrument and thorough content analysis of respondents' comments) indicate that findings can be generalised to the wider population of DSNs. They can also be generalised to CNSs working in areas other than diabetes, because the DSN role follows the principles cited in the literature as part of the wider CNS population.

This study provides tangible evidence not only for the clarification of the DSN role performance and role components, but also for the wider context in which the implementation and development of this role are undertaken. This research project, the first national survey in the UK to examine the overall role of the DSN, was a strength of the present study and stimulated respondents' interest.

Despite the strengths of this study, a number of limitations were also inherent. Although the response rate (51.2%) is representative of the wider population of DSNs, it is lower compared to other quantitative studies documented in the nursing literature. Other limitations regarding this study related to the instrument used to collect data. The research instrument utilised in the present study explored the following concepts derived from role theory and related to the DSN role:

- Personal characteristics and skills
- Work setting and organisational factors
- Role development
- Role performance.

A previously tested instrument by Hamric and Taylor (1989) was adopted for the measurement of DSN role development. This proved very useful in describing this complex process and eliciting data regarding the factors that facilitate and inhibit role implementation. Three scales were developed by the researcher based on the CNS and DSN literature to measure the remaining concepts. To establish its reliability and validity, the instrument was reviewed by a panel of seven experts and pre-tested in a pilot study. Data obtained from the main study were analysed using an exploratory factor analysis, with maximum likelihood extraction which identified the underlying dimensions of each scale and the variables salient to each dimension. Moreover, this statistical method allowed findings to be projected to a wider population. A high internal consistency was found for the scales developed for the purpose of this study. Following this procedure, an instrument with strong content validity and reliability was developed to measure the role-related parameters of the DSN.

Despite its statistical strength, a number of limitations were present. Considering the multifaceted nature of the DSN role, it would be unrealistic to assert that this instrument captured all the dimensions combined within the role. As this was the first empirical utilisation of this instrument, further investigation is required in order to confirm its high reliability and to establish its scientific rigour and validity.

7.7 Study implications for CNS practice

A number of issues prevailed from the comprehensive exploration of the role of DSNs in the UK and the factors that influence the successful development and performance of their role. On the basis of the results of the present study, recommendations are made relevant to each DSN role concept explored in the previous chapters of this book.

7.7.1 Educational (academic) qualifications

- A nationally agreed course at postgraduate level needs to be organised for the preparation of DSNs. It is suggested that this course is at Master's level and lasts at least one academic year. It can be designed for the general population of CNSs and does not need to focus specifically on diabetes. It must provide nurses with advanced knowledge covering the main areas and components of their multifaceted role.
- Master's level of education should be the entry criterion for CNS practice for newly employed practitioners. Similarly, existing CNSs should undertake further formal education at Master's level and it is important that nursing administration supports them in this direction.

7.7.2 Role development: developmental phases

- Educators need to understand the process of role development in order to provide CNSs with adequate preparation for their expanded role.
- Both CNSs and nurse administrators need to have a clear understanding of the CNS role in order to set realistic expectations and targets for role performance. This understanding can offer guidance for role implementation for novice CNSs, who may not have the skills to divide their time and effort among the many components and activities of their role.

- It is vital that guidelines and expectations for each level of the role development exist in written form and be realistic and achievable.

7.7.3 Qualifications, personal characteristics and skills

- The present study revealed that personal characteristics and skills of the DSN present the greatest predictor for his/her role performance. Therefore, emphasis must be given to the enhancement of these characteristics. Teaching these skills and strategies to enhance personal attributes must be incorporated into the academic educational preparation of CNSs, or provided as in-service training.
- CNSs need to understand that role-related skills, attributes and competence are enhanced through role development and progression through the phases of their role. Therefore, they should have realistic self-expectations and set goals when entering the role. CNSs also need to understand that continuous update and education are crucial in maintaining and increasing their competence in their area of practice.

7.7.4 Work setting and organisational factors

- Findings of this study suggested that the DSN role does not exist in isolation and is greatly influenced by factors deriving from work settings. It is crucial for nursing administration and other health professionals to realise that they will not benefit from the CNS practice unless they provide them with support, understanding and recognition.
- It is important that CNSs realise that if others do not understand the benefits of their role they will not support it but will rather try to eliminate it. Urgent clarification of the CNS role at a national level is, therefore, crucial to the survival and success of this role.

7.7.5 Role performance: role components and activities

- Greater involvement of CNSs in research activities is required if their role is to be an integrated one. Their research skills must be developed through graduate programmes.
- It is important to note that, although all the role components are essential, the time allotted to each depends on the CNS job description and work setting, as well as the expectations imposed on the CNS by the administration, peers, other nursing staff and health professionals; and time allotted to clients' immediate needs must also be taken into account. Priorities and realistic expectations for performance need to be set. CNSs should realise that they do not have to become 'all things to all people', as this may result in them feeling frustrated, anxious and overwhelmed.

7.8 Recommendations and conclusion

7.8.1 Recommendations for practising nurses and administrators

The present study indicated that the CNS role is complex and flexible, and does not exist in isolation. Support and understanding from all significant parties are vital if the CNS role is to be successful. It is, therefore, apparent that role clarification should be a priority, if not the most important objective, in the process of role implementation. If others do not understand the nature, benefits and potential use of the role, they will not accept CNSs as advanced practitioners; rather they will view them as intruders and try to eliminate the CNS role. This can be achieved by developing a clear, understandable and well-written job description. It should be concise and to the point but long enough to state exactly who the CNS is, what he or she provides in the particular setting and to whom he or she is accountable. The CNS's role responsibilities should be determined in close collaboration and discussion with the manager and the CNS. The job description should be disseminated and explained to all health professionals that cooperate with CNSs in order to achieve their maximum support and best use of this role. Clarification of the role to patients and their families is equally important.

CNSs have an advanced level of practice and knowledge. Retaining CNSs in the clinical area means that they should be provided with equal opportunities for role advancement with teachers and administrators. The challenge, therefore, for administrators in collaboration with CNSs should be the development of an appropriate promotional system, within the boundaries of clinical practice, which offers the ongoing stimulation that expert CNSs need to maintain growth. With regard to the UK setting, consideration should be given to the grading criteria for specialist nursing in order to reflect the appropriate level of role advancement of each CNS. The implementation of the *NHS Knowledge and Skills Framework* (Department of Health, 2004) for nursing and midwifery can prove valuable in eliminating the existing inequalities across the UK regarding the different levels of the CNS practice. In addition, monetary recognition is the most tangible reward for clinical excellence and, thus, it should keep pace with that of other staff of comparable education and experience within the institution. Opportunities and funding for further education and outside professional activities should be provided to all CNSs.

Nurse administrators, other health professionals and CNSs themselves need to realise that CNSs cannot be 'everything to all people' and undertake all role components and activities simultaneously. Objectives and role responsibilities have to be prioritised according to patients' and health professionals' immediate needs, as well as according to the available resources.

7.8.2 Recommendations for nurse educators

The present study revealed that CNSs require an advanced level of educational preparation in order to successfully undertake their multifaceted role. Educators need to understand the complex nature and the process of development and implementation of the role and provide CNSs with adequate preparation for their expanded role. In the UK at present, different educational programmes are available which provide varied levels of preparation for the CNS. Therefore, an emergent need exists for the development and implementation of a unique national course at Master's level which lasts at least one academic year.

It is suggested that the curriculum of the CNS course includes modules which cover all the areas and components of the CNS role, namely clinical practice, teaching, consultation, management, leadership, and research skills. The design of this programme should comply with the standards for specialist education and practice set by the Nursing and Midwifery Council (United Kingdom Central Council, 1994). Topics such as theoretical foundations of nursing, healthcare policy and finance, ethical decision-making, role development process, organisational theory, health promotion and disease prevention are significant to the CNS role and should also be included in the content of the Master's degree curriculum. In addition, this programme should include modules which enhance the CNS's personal characteristics and communication, collaboration and interpersonal skills. It is important that this course is provided in different universities across the country in order to eliminate the accessibility constraints for CNS candidates. Alternatively, distance learning and web-based materials may be developed.

7.8.3 Recommendations for future research

The theoretical framework underpinning the study combined six concepts related to the CNS role (*Chapter 2*), of which four were examined in this study. Further exploration of the remaining two concepts, role expectations and role stress, is required in order to identify their association with the CNS role. The present study revealed that CNSs in the UK reported a similar process of role development to that of CNSs in North America (Hamric and Taylor, 1989). It would be beneficial to explore whether this role development model can be similarly applied to CNSs working in the UK, in areas other than diabetes. Hamric and Taylor (1989) tested the model with CNSs from a wide range of specialities in the USA. Testing with other groups of advanced nurse practitioners could identify whether these follow patterns of role development similar to that of CNSs.

This study was the first empirical evidence suggesting that role performance of CNSs is interrelated with their personal characteristics and skills, their role development, and work setting and organisational factors. Further research involving other groups of CNSs is required in order to verify the reliability and generalisability of findings in the wider population of CNSs and the value of the theoretical framework in exploring the CNS role. Investigation of whether the theoretical framework derived from role theory is useful in guiding the exploration of the role of other groups of advanced nurse practitioners and general nurses would also be valuable.

8

A perspective of the role of the diabetes specialist nurse from Greece

8.1 Introduction

From the discussion in the previous chapters of this book, it is concluded that the DSN role has been clearly established in the UK. Its development has followed the general patterns of clinical specialist nursing and presents a close resemblance to the role of the CNS in North America.

Diabetes nursing as a clinical speciality has not yet been implemented in Greece. The nursing care of people with diabetes is undertaken by general nurses, whose qualifications and responsibilities are varied, and their role has not yet been documented. The feasibility of implementing the DSN role in the Greek healthcare system is explored in this chapter. Five focus groups were conducted to explore opinions of physicians and nurses working in diabetes centres in Athens, and of patients with diabetes.

The first part of the chapter describes the research design and methods adopted to explore the perspective of the DSN role in Greece. The advantages and any potential obstacles in the process of implementing the DSN role, and the identification of strategies to overcome these, are presented in the second part. The results have been illustrated by a wide range of comments and/or discussions. It was believed that a better understanding of perceptions can be obtained through respondents' own words (original data) rather than the researcher's interpretation of these.

8.2 Review of the literature

In contrast to the UK, diabetes care in Greece is principally undertaken in the hospital setting, which also provides primary care services through outpatient departments. Following the St Vincent Declaration in 1989 regarding targets of diabetes care, the Greek Government undertook enhanced measures to institute thirteen diabetes centres in public hospitals affiliated to universities. There are ten in Athens, two in Thessaloniki and one in Patra (Bartsokas, 1999). Physician diabetologists, nurses (including health visitors) and dieticians are full-time members of the multidisciplinary healthcare teams operating in most of these centres. Other physicians (nephrologists, ophthalmologists) and health professionals (social workers, psychologists) may work part-time in, or liaise with, these teams when needed. A major constraint in the functioning of diabetes teams in Greece is the rare, if not absent, community-hospital coordination.

In addition to the affiliated centres, diabetes care is also provided by 62 diabetes outpatient clinics in public hospitals across Greece (Halvatsiotis *et al*, 2000). These clinics are either fully dedicated to diabetes or provide part-time services in diabetes (three days per week). The service provided varies according to the following factors: geographical location, access to specialised diabetes care, and qualifications of the healthcare teams. These may or may not be multidisciplinary. Research is an important task for health professionals working in diabetes centres, along with their primary role in the care and education of patients and their families, and health personnel training (Bartsokas, 1999). However, the nursing input into research and staff training is limited.

Almost fifteen years ago, the Greek Department of Health recommended that each diabetes centre and diabetes outpatients clinic should appoint at least one qualified nurse educated at first-degree level who, among other nursing responsibilities, would undertake comprehensive education of patients with diabetes and their carers (Hellenic DoH, 1990). However, a large proportion of nurses currently working in diabetes care, particularly in outpatient clinics, has only received a two-year nursing education. Their responsibilities are limited to the provision of routine direct care activities and clerical work.

Diabetes nursing as a clinical speciality has not yet been implemented in Greece. The nursing care of people with diabetes is undertaken by general nurses, whose qualifications and responsibilities are varied. Diabetes care is mainly undertaken in the hospital setting, which also provides primary care services. The role of nursing in the provision of diabetes care in Greece remains vague, and the responsibilities and qualifications of nurses working in this area vary from setting to setting.

Even though Greece has the second highest prevalence of type 2 diabetes in Europe (International Diabetes Federation, 2000), there is no literature documenting the provision of diabetes care and the role of the nurse working in this area. Moreover, the role of the DSN has not yet been introduced in the Greek healthcare sector and there is very limited literature in Greek relating to this role (Lemonidou, 1999; Llahana and Gerogianni, 2003).

Due to the unavailability of information in this area, a qualitative study was undertaken aiming to:

- Provide information regarding the practice, responsibilities and qualifications of nurses working in diabetes care in Greece, and
- Explore opinions of health professionals and patients with diabetes regarding the feasibility of implementing the role of the DSN in Greece, guided by the UK model of the DSN role described in the previous chapters of this book.

8.3 Design and methods

8.3.1 Why use focus group interviews?

The focus group interview was considered the most appropriate qualitative method, as the main objective was to obtain a diversity of beliefs and opinions regarding the feasibility of implementing the DSN role in a new setting. Clarke (1999: p395) noted that:

> *'The purpose of focus groups is to develop an understanding of perceptions, beliefs, attitudes and experience, and to explore the context in which these were formed.'*

According to McDaniel and Bach (1996), the group interaction stimulates the discussion that provides the researcher with the opportunity to collect data and insights, and which does not occur with other data collection methods. Group members influence each other with their comments, and participants may form opinions after considering the views of others.

Focus group interviews can be used for collecting data relating to a wide range of purposes. The relevance of this method to the objectives of the present study was supported by the following applications of focus groups. Firstly, they are useful when existing knowledge of a subject is inadequate or non-existent (Powell and Single, 1996). As already noted, the practice of nurses working in diabetes care in Greece has not been previously documented. Moreover, the concept of the DSN role has not been introduced in the Greek setting. Secondly, this method can help to identify key issues in a new field and elicit participants' perceptions, insights and attitudes toward a particular topic or a proposed change, as well as to generate hypotheses relating to this topic (Jackson, 1998b). A description of the role of diabetes nurses in Greece was the aim throughout this study. The main objective, however, was to explore opinions of physicians, nurses and patients regarding the feasibility of implementing the DSN role in the Greek healthcare system guided by the UK model explored in the previous chapters. This study also aimed to identify any potential advantages and constraints to the implementation of the DSN role in the Greek setting. Focus group interviews are useful in providing data when preparing for changes in policy or for achieving the implementation of a policy (Robinson, 1999). The ultimate aim of this study, to provide evidence that could impact on the implementation of the DSN role in Greece, was a further rationale for the use of this method.

Focus group interviews provide a wide variety of views and a large amount of participant interaction about a topic in a relatively short time. Moreover, they are low-cost and relatively easy to conduct, compared to other methods (Al-Zaru, 2001; Jackson, 1998n; Parahoo, 1997; Stewart and Shamdasani, 1990). The use of focus groups is not without limitations. As in other qualitative methods, results are not generalisable due to the small sample size and specificity of data to a particular context (Clarke, 1999).

8.3.2 Planning the focus group interviews

Reiskin (1992) suggested four phases when using focus group interviews: planning, conducting the interviews, analysing the data obtained, and reporting the findings. The following agenda of questions was designed to elicit information from the focus group sessions according to the objectives of this study:

1. What are the responsibilities and practice of nurses working in diabetes care in Greece?
2. How do health professionals and patients perceive the role of the DSN?
3. What are the advantages of implementing the DSN role in Greece?
4. What constraints and obstacles, if any, exist in the implementation of the DSN role in the Greek healthcare system?
5. What do health professionals and patients in Greece perceive as the required qualifications for a DSN? and

6. What pathway should be followed for the successful implementation of the diabetes nursing speciality in the Greek healthcare system?

These questions were reviewed for content validity by three expert researchers. As questions were initially formulated in English and then translated, one of the experts, a native Greek speaker, confirmed that the meaning of questions remained the same after they had been translated into Greek. Moreover, the guideline questions were pre-tested in a pilot focus group interview.

8.3.3 Sample identification and recruitment

A purposive sampling, by involving a conscious selection of individuals (Al-Zaru, 2001), was adopted. This has been defined by Arber (1993) as the broad sampling method for studies that are aimed at a wider understanding of social processes and actions. The inclusion criteria for participants were physician diabetologists and qualified nurses working in diabetes centres in Athens, as well as patients with diabetes. In order to obtain a diversity of opinions, it was decided to arrange groups of: a) physicians only; b) nurses only; c) physicians and nurses; and d) physicians, nurses and patients.

In Greece, there are thirteen diabetes centres operating in public hospitals affiliated to universities, which are located in three major cities (Bartsokas, 1999). Seven diabetes centres, located in Athens (capital of Greece), were involved. Of these, two provide care exclusively to children (paediatric hospitals) and five to adults. Managers of the diabetes centres were informed of the objectives of the study, and were asked for permission to conduct the focus group interviews and to provide a study sample. The number of physicians employed in these diabetes centres varied from three to six, and that of nurses from one to three. Four patients attending one of the seven diabetes centres were invited to participate in the study after ethical permission had been obtained from the manager of the centre. The final selected sample number was 37 participants: nineteen physicians, fourteen nurses, and four patients with diabetes (*Table 8.1*).

8.3.4 Introducing the research topic

Prior to inviting participants to attend the focus group interviews, the researcher visited the diabetes centres selected for the study and had the opportunity of meeting the majority of physicians and nurses. It was found that only a very limited number of them were familiar with the DSN role. Moreover, focus group interviews in Greece are rarely used in health research. It was, therefore, crucial for participants involved in the study to become familiar with the characteristics of this role in order to be able to express their opinions and attitudes. The researcher presented a seminar for all participants which aimed to remedy this shortcoming. The following areas were addressed:

- How is a CNS defined and what are the components and activities constituting their role performance?
- What is the role of the DSN?
- What is the purpose of focus group interviews and how are they conducted?

8.3.5 Scientific rigour of focus group interviews

Findings from focus group interviews are not replicable and cannot be generalised. In contrast to quantitative studies, the reliability of data collection from focus group interviews cannot be determined through statistical procedures and psychometric tests. McDaniel and Bach (1996: p54) consider that reliability

> *'…can only be determined by careful review of the description of the procedures used to select subjects, the methods of observing and recording, and the process of data analysis.'*

They also maintain that focus group research should be evaluated on the basis of trustworthiness, which is composed of credibility, dependability, confirmability, and transferability.

8.3.5.1 Credibility

Credibility is similar to validity used in quantitative research and considers the truth-value of findings and their ability to faithfully interpret participants' experiences (Al-Zaru, 2001). According to McDaniel and Bach (1996), credibility can be enhanced through the investigator's prolonged engagement with this research method. It can also be enhanced by requesting feedback from participants about the accuracy of the researcher's data interpretation. As noted earlier, the researcher undertook extensive preparation to enhance her skills in conducting the focus group interviews and analysing and presenting the results. In addition, five participants compared the analyses and the transcripts of the interviews, and verified the content validity of the data.

8.3.5.2 Transferability

McDaniel and Bach (1996) defined transferability as reflecting the ability of findings of a study to be applicable to another similar context, group or setting. However, transferability does not denote generalisability, and it is inappropriate to project findings to a wider population. Transferability in this study was enhanced by providing a detailed description of the data from which results were drawn.

8.3.5.3 Dependability

Dependability allows other researchers to follow logically the processes and procedures that the investigator used in a study (McDaniel and Bach, 1996). In the present study, the research procedure was reviewed by two researchers with expertise in focus group interviews. A third researcher examined the translated questions and confirmed that they 'fitted' into the Greek setting.

8.3.5.4 Confirmability

Confirmability is achieved when another independent investigator, who follows the researcher's decisions and procedure in conducting the study, reaches similar conclusions about the data (McDaniel and Bach, 1996). In this study, the researcher followed the suggestions made by Polit and Hungler (1999) and described, explained and justified each stage of the process of conducting focus group interviews and of analysing and presenting the results.

8.3.5.5 Pre-testing the research questions

The guideline questions were pre-tested with a pilot group of five participants (two physicians and three nurses) who did not work exclusively in the diabetes field, but provided care to patients with diabetes in their practice. A prerequisite for participants attending this pilot interview, as for all the other focus group interviews, was that they attended the seminar presentation described above. Minor ambiguities relating to the questions and their wording were identified and clarified. The time frame for each question (the allocation of adequate time for covering each question without exceeding the agreed overall time of the session) was also tested.

8.3.6 Data collection

There is a consensus that the number of participants in the focus group should be between four and ten people (Clarke, 1999; Jackson, 1998b; Stewart and Shamdasani, 1990). However, McLafferty (2004) suggested that the group should be large enough to allow adequate participation of all members and small enough to avoid the risk of providing similar coverage to that of a one-to-one interview.

Five focus group interviews were conducted in this study, although six had been planned initially. The selected sample and the number of respondents for each focus group session are presented in *Table 8.1.* One focus group was composed of two nurses and, although the reliability of data obtained from a group of two participants is questionable (Kitzinger and Barbour, 1999), it was found that they provided information significant to the study.

All participants were contacted by telephone one or two days in advance and reminded about the forthcoming focus group session. The overall number of respondents was nineteen (*Table 8.1*).

Table 8.1 Selected sample, number of participants agreeing to attend the focus group interviews and number of those who actually attended

Focus group number	Selected sample of participants	Respondents agreeing to participate	Respondents attending the focus group interviews
1	3 physicians 2 nurses 4 patients	3 physicians 2 nurses 3 patients	2 physicians 1 nurse 2 patients
2	5 physicians 3 nurses	3 physicians 3 nurses	1 physician 3 nurses
3	5 physicians 2 nurses	3 physicians 2 nurses	2 physicians 2 nurses
4	2 nurses (paediatric diabetes ctr) 3 nurses (adult diabetes ctr)	2 nurses (paediatric diabetes ctr) 3 nurses (adult diabetes ctr)	2 nurses (paediatric diabetes ctr) 2 nurses (adult diabetes ctr)
5	2 nurses	2 nurses	2 nurses
6*	6 physicians	4 physicians	1 physician*
Total	37	27	19

* *As only one participant attended this session, data obtained were not included in the study*

The discussion in the focus groups was guided by the agenda of questions described earlier. The interviews were conducted in Greek and each session lasted approximately one hour. The researcher obtained the participants' agreement to tape-record the interviews. Confidentiality was also considered and, although this is difficult to achieve among the members of the same group (Kitzinger and Barbour, 1999), the researcher assured participants that she would be the only person having access to the recorded interviews. Moreover, participants were informed that no reference would be made to their identity or the name of the diabetes centre when the results were reported.

8.3.7 Data analysis

Kitzinger and Barbour (1999: p16) stressed that:

> '*...the researcher needs to reference the group context. This means starting from an analysis of groups rather than individuals and striking a balance between looking at the picture provided by the group as a whole and recognizing the operation of individual "voices" within it.*'

Thus, as the present study emphasised, interaction between participants' data was analysed at both a group and an individual level, using the guidelines of Reiskin (1992), McDaniel and Bach (1996), and Kitzinger and Barbour (1999):

- The tape-recorded interviews were transcribed verbatim immediately after the session in combination with the additional field notes of the moderator and those relating to the non-verbal communication. The transcripts were then reviewed along with the tapes and notes to confirm the accuracy of transcription.
- Transcripts were read carefully in order to identify the sections relevant to the research questions. A coding system for major topics and ideas was developed. Following this, each transcript was read independently and organised into categories, which were examined for themes, patterns, similar words and context. Data were organised into different categories according to the guideline questions.

After this analysis, the original transcripts were translated into English. Al-Zaru (2001) stressed that several issues should be considered in relation to the translation of transcripts which may have particular implications for the quality of data. Twinn (1998: p657) identified some:

> '*The first of these relates to the translation of words for which there is no true equivalent in the source language...* [In addition] *...the influence of grammatical style is another finding that affects the quality of data.*'

Although the structure of sentences and grammar rules differ substantially between Greek and English, the researcher translated the interviews as literally as possible. However, different metaphors and idioms used by respondents were translated according to their equivalent meaning in English. A linguistics expert in both Greek and English examined the translations to confirm that the meanings remained unchanged.

English versions were subjected to data analysis in a similar procedure to the original analysis. The same themes and conceptual categories emerged, indicating that translation had not influenced the originality of the data. After coding and conceptual categorisation, the data were systematically explored to generate meaning (Coffey and Atkinson, 1996). At the final stage, analysis involved drawing together and comparing discussion of similar themes. The relationship of these to the variation between individuals and groups was then examined (Kitzinger and Barbour, 1999).

The results obtained from the analysis are presented and discussed according to the guideline questions for the focus group interviews.

8.4 Results

Although the data obtained from the focus group interviews have been coded into theoretical themes and categories, the results have been illustrated by a wide range of respondents' comments and interactions.

8.4.1 Responsibilities and practice of diabetes nurses in Greece

As in all areas of nursing, in diabetes the job description for nurses in Greece varies from hospital to hospital and is at the discretion of each institution and/or nursing management. A wide variation was found between the responsibilities of nurses working in the diabetes centres included in the present study. The majority of respondents were involved in direct care, education and a limited number of consultation activities. However, there were nurses who had mainly clerical responsibilities and whose clinical responsibilities were limited to basic procedures.

The following responses were given by nurses participating in two different focus groups to the question 'Please describe briefly your job responsibilities and tasks in this Diabetes Centre':

Focus group 5

> *'...We prepare the file for each patient by filling in their personal details, their height and weight... If we see that someone has hypoglycaemia whilst waiting to see the doctor, we offer them something sweet to drink or eat...'* (Nurse A)
>
> *'...we can give patients the insulin injection, for example, when they are here if they cannot do it themselves...'* (Nurse B)
>
> *'...we demonstrate the use of insulin pens and explain the injection technique to those patients who are starting on insulin...'* (Nurse A)
>
> *'...where to inject his insulin, how to store insulin, and things like that. That is in general terms what we do...'* (Nurse B)
>
> *'...if doctors need something else they will ask us. Like for example "Please advise Mrs X on how to contact the dietician..."; things like that...'* (Nurse A)

At the other extreme, however, as illustrated in the following example, another respondent reported undertaking most of the activities constituting the DSN role:

Focus group 4

> *'...I undertake all the education of the child diagnosed with diabetes, from the moment he is admitted to the hospital until the day he goes home. This education*

> *includes everything that a child and his family should know regarding self-management of diabetes. Moreover, there is follow-up education and an effort to coordinate with other team members. Furthermore, I am involved in research and in the education of health professionals and students, including also formal education in diabetes at the University of Nursing. …we do not have the authority to prescribe. In most cases, I fill in the prescription and the doctor signs it. There is also telephone support in the Centre and, at the same time, I have provided parents and patients with my private telephone number, where they can contact me at any time in case of emergency.'* (Nurse A)

This diversity was also reflected in the nursing education and other qualifications of nurses participating in the present study. Of the twelve nurses, three had received a two-year nursing education and nine held a first degree in nursing. Of the three who held a Master's degree, one was undertaking doctoral education at the time of the study.

8.4.2 Perceptions regarding the DSN role

All respondents in the present study perceived the DSN role as essential in the care of people with diabetes and emphasised the importance of its implementation in the Greek healthcare system. However, the majority saw the DSN functioning as a diabetes educator rather than having a role that incorporated all the role components identified in the literature. Nurses, however, did not see this role component as simply relieving physicians of the need to educate patients. They considered the DSN to be the most appropriate person to undertake, as one nurse noted, the 'painstaking long-term process of education'. Moreover, they perceived the DSN as the health professional responsible for the long-term follow-up care of patients.

Patients, on the other hand, expressed the need for support and for someone to be able to listen to their concerns. They referred to the physicians' inability to devote the necessary time to patients, and their approach which:

> '*…does not make you feel comfortable and open up. When they* [physicians] *speak, they do not use "my language", as a nurse would do. They use a lot of jargon, and I am already at home before I can put my head around what they have said, so no chance to ask for explanations'* (Patient A; Focus group).

Patients felt more comfortable approaching the nurse than any other member of the team but, at the same time, expressed the need for nurses to be appropriately qualified in order to be able to 'stand by the patient'.

8.4.3 Perceptions regarding the components and activities of the DSN role

As reported earlier, findings with respect to the DSN role performance in the UK were introduced to respondents in the seminar presentation preceding the focus group interviews. A list of the components and activities constituting the DSN role performance was distributed to participants. This was identical to the activities included in the DSN role performance explored in *Chapter 6*. Respondents in the focus groups were asked to comment on the DSN role and its relevance to the Greek healthcare setting. The following five role components were explored: expert practice, education, consultation, research, and leadership.

8.4.3.1 Expert practitioner

Respondents perceived this role component as an important aspect of the DSN role. All the groups emphasised the importance of providing support to patients and their families over the telephone. They reported that in Greece patients have no access to specialised support in case of emergency at times other than the morning shift. For this reason, they believed that a 24-hour help line is crucial. One important activity which nurses do not undertake in the Greek setting is that of home visits. Respondents reported that the provision of this service is essential in the absence of hospital-community coordination currently existing, and could be undertaken by a hospital-based DSN. One nurse who had previously undertaken home visits, but had to stop due to time constraints and the increase in patient caseload, commented:

> *'This activity was a very important aspect of my role. You enter the patient's home and you see how he lives, how he behaves, you come close to him... He will talk to you about his psychological problems, his family affairs; you see his living environment.'* (Nurse; Focus group 1)

On the other hand, almost all physicians opposed the idea of the DSN undertaking advanced specialised care activities. They considered that a nurse could not acquire the appropriate knowledge to undertake activities such as prescribing diabetes-related medications, ordering laboratory tests, and providing specialised care to patients with complex physical problems. They believed that such activities '...presuppose certain medical knowledge, which can only be acquired by attending medical school'. Similarly, as illustrated in the following interaction, many nurses did not believe they would be able to reach such an advanced level of practice to function autonomously:

> *'I can tell the doctor my opinion, but I cannot make the final decision because I do not have this knowledge...'.* (Nurse A; Focus group 2)
>
> *'...The DSN can certainly have the first contact with the patient, but she should then transfer the information to the doctor.* (Physician B; Focus group 2)

8.4.3.2 Educator

The importance of the DSN functioning as an educator was highlighted by all respondents in this study and this role component was perceived as the main aspect of the DSN role. Respondents emphasised the role of the nurse in the education of patients and their families, particularly in group teaching.

Respondents perceived the involvement of the DSN in informing the public about diabetes as vital, in order to solve the problem of 'stigmatisation' that patients with diabetes face in Greece. Diabetes education for school staff and pupils was also highlighted. However, one paediatric nurse who provided education to schools reported that this could often be difficult to achieve. She noted:

> *'Many parents do not allow me to inform the school staff that this child has diabetes... They do not want others to know that their child is "diabetic". Not only does*

> *this place me in a great dilemma, but also children often end up in hospital'.* (Nurse A; Focus group 4)

Respondents' opinion about the provision of education to medical staff by the DSN varied. Although more than half of respondents believed that a DSN can educate physicians regarding diabetes issues, many others did not. Two physicians reported that the DSN should only be able to provide education to physicians on technical matters, for example, injection techniques and use of insulin pens. One commented:

> *'A nurse, no matter how educated she is, cannot provide education to physicians... Only the medical staff provide education to the nursing staff, not the other way around!'* (Physician B; Focus group 1)

Similarly, two nurses felt that '...a doctor would never accept my opinion!'. They believed that the medically-dominated health system that exists at present in many hospitals expects the nurse to be at a 'lower level than the doctor'. Patients also agreed with this, with one commenting:

> *'It is a question of mentality that, in Greece, the nurse still has a different image than that of the nurse abroad. ...I do not think that a doctor would accept to be educated by a nurse, even if she is a specialist in her field'.* (Patient B; Focus group 1)

8.4.3.3 Consultant

Respondents considered that nurses should act as consultants only to enable patients and their families to cope with the immediate crisis of diagnosis and long-term adjustments in life style. The need for this was particularly highlighted by patients, who felt more comfortable approaching the nurse than any other member of the healthcare team.

Respondents perceived that an important aspect of the DSN role in consultation was in relation to the organisation of care, i.e. setting standards, development and implementation of policies, protocols and care pathways. However, they believed that the present structure of the healthcare system in Greece does not provide nurses with the authority to undertake such activities. The following comments were made:

> *'Concerning the facts in Greece, these all* [consultation activities] *sound a bit funny. Here we are unable to communicate properly within the same hospital, let alone in a region or even more in the whole country!'* (Physician A; Focus group 1)

> *'DSNs could really have a valuable say on what is happening, but under the present situation, nobody would listen to what they say. Their advice would have no value, if they do not have the authority...'* (Physician A; Focus group 3)

It was also felt that the DSN could have a valuable role in the organisation of patient support groups. Some respondents reported that they had organised support groups, but these lacked consistent planning and coordination. Moreover, as this was not included in their job description, their input into these was purely voluntary.

8.4.3.4 Researcher

Respondents perceived the involvement of the nurse in research activities in the clinical area as a 'luxury'. Although two nurse respondents were involved in research, this was a component of their academic educational programme (MSc, Doctorate). The identified reasons for this were the lack of research skills of nurses, time constraints, and '...the fact that the nurse is not viewed as an equal member of the healthcare team'. Many respondents believed that, even if the DSN role were implemented in Greece, the only way for them to be involved in research would be in cooperation with the University of Nursing. However, they stressed that, '...there are so many things that the DSN will have to do that research will seem "unreachable"'.

Physicians in one focus group believed that nursing education cannot provide the appropriate skills for undertaking research studies, which they construed as purely clinical research. One commented:

> *'...Fine! Research is also what you do* [addressing the researcher], *but in Greece, in the clinical area, the meaning of research is completely different. It refers to clinical studies, and this is what we expect when we say research. I do not think that a nurse has the background to undertake such activities'.* (Physician B; Focus group 1)

8.4.3.5 Manager/leader

Respondents reported that the only activity in the manager/leader role component relevant to the Greek setting would be the DSN participation in identifying gaps in the diabetes care services; the remaining were viewed as irrelevant. Respondents believed that, in Greece, this component could not be incorporated in the role of the DSN. They noted that the structure and organisation of the healthcare system do not provide the nurse with the authority to 'make her voice heard'. This is illustrated in the following interaction:

> *'The advice of the DSN would be valuable if accepted, because they are the professionals who really know the needs of this field. They should be able to say, for example: "We have come across with this problem. You should provide funds for home visits, which is very important".'* (Physician A; Focus group 3)
>
> *'...Yes, I agree! The same applies to the input of hiring nursing staff in the diabetes centre, because the DSN is the most appropriate person to assess this. While if we need a new nurse, they will employ the first one from the "waiting for employment" list. This is unfortunately how the administration system works here!.'* (Nurse B; Focus group 3)

8.4.4 Advantages of implementing the DSN role in Greece

Respondents perceived the improvement in patient care as the greatest advantage to implementing the DSN role in Greece. They commented that the DSN would be able to monitor the condition of patients more frequently than physicians, and thus improve their metabolic control and reduce the frequency of complications.

Most physicians agreed with this perception and noted that an additional advantage would be for patients to have an appropriately qualified person able to listen to and discuss their concerns. Similarly, patients felt that they would be able to talk with greater ease with a DSN rather than a physician:

> '…*I want information about everything! But when I see 30 people waiting to see the doctor, I think: "I should discuss my most urgent concerns and better forget about the rest!"…I would not, however, worry if I knew that after the doctor I would see the DSN who could explain me everything I want to know*' (Patient A; Focus group 1)

Another advantage identified to implementing the DSN role in Greece was related to the reduction of treatment cost for diabetes. Respondents considered that DSNs would have a greater impact than physicians on the appropriate follow-up of patients, thus reducing the long-term diabetes complications, which, as one physician noted, '…is what we are mostly battling with.'

Patients with complications usually have to be admitted to hospital and, as in Greece there are no community facilities for continued follow-up care, they have to stay in hospital until fully recovered. Respondents noted that if DSNs were appointed in hospitals, patients could be discharged earlier, as the DSN could undertake their follow-up care at home. Therefore, the cost of treatment would decrease substantially. Moreover, they perceived the establishment of community-hospital cooperation and the DSN as a link between the two settings as crucial to the improvement of patient care. This is illustrated in the following interaction:

> '*It would be helpful if every hospital would establish cooperation with a number of health centres in the community…*' (Physician A; Focus group 1)

> '*We could have a DSN in our hospital who could cooperate with the health centre and provide care for patients with complex problems. She could also train nurses there who, at present, do not have the appropriate diabetes skills…*' (Nurse; Focus group 1)

The final advantage identified by respondents related to nursing as a profession. This was particularly highlighted by nurses who believed that not only would the implementation of the DSN role advance their knowledge and skills, but it would also enhance the status of nurses in the healthcare team. They believed that the title of DSN would provide them with the authority to undertake advanced responsibilities and be recognised as an advanced practitioner. One nurse commented characteristically:

> '…*at present, unfortunately, all nursing staff do ostensibly the same job, regardless of qualifications or education. That is to say, I, with a Master's degree, have the same responsibilities as an assistant nurse who has only received two years of nursing education. When, however, the patient has had a bad experience with this nurse, how is it possible for him to trust my expertise since I am also a nurse? Whereas, when the DSN role is formalised and the responsibilities are clarified, then the patient will be able to see the difference and trust the DSN. This will also be the case for other health professionals, particularly for the medical staff.*' (Nurse B; Focus group 4)

8.4.5 Constraints and obstacles to the implementation of the DSN role in Greece

The fourth question was:

- What constraints and obstacles, if any, exist in the implementation of the DSN role in the Greek healthcare system?

A range of constraints and obstacles were identified which often overlapped and/or were interrelated. However, for the purposes of this discussion they are presented separately.

8.4.5.1 Status quo of nursing administration and employment of nursing staff

The greatest obstacle to the implementation of the DSN role in the Greek healthcare system was related to the status quo of nursing management and the structure of employment for nursing staff. In Greece, the nursing administrators of public hospitals, or of particular departments within these hospitals, do not have the authority to select their nursing staff. Rather, graduate nurses enter a 'waiting for employment' list and are then appointed through the Ministry of Health. Hospitals indicate the number of nurses they need and the Ministry of Health selects from the list, for example, the first twenty nurses. Nurses can select the hospital of choice but not the area or speciality of employment. Nursing positions are announced for general nurses, independent of their special qualifications or job preferences. Nurses are then allocated to departments according to the need, or at the discretion of nursing administration.

This constraint is also related to the 'rotation system' used by nursing administration in most hospitals. For example, a nurse working in the diabetes centre of a hospital can be transferred to work in the cardiology unit in order to cover the needs of this department, as funds are not available to employ new staff. This constraint was closely associated with the shortages of nursing staff, and as one respondent commented:

> '*...nursing administration has no other choice but cover the immediate needs of each department. It is justifiable to move staff around when there is no possibility of employing new nurses*'. (Nurse B; Focus group 2)

This system results in many nurses not being able to apply their acquired specialisation and skills in a particular area. As one respondent noted, '...it all goes wasted and you have to start from the beginning.' Because of the above constraints, many nurses reported being reluctant to undertake further education or training. One nurse commented: 'Why should I waste my time? Who guarantees me that after I finish or even sometime in the future I will be able to work in this area?'

In addition, respondents reported that further qualifications or specialisation in a particular area were not always recognised by administration. Nurses were not granted promotion, reward or any other privileges, and were not guaranteed employment in their area of expertise. Moreover, as illustrated below, nurses reported great difficulties in obtaining time off to attend seminars or study days:

> '*...If we, let us say, need to leave one hour earlier to attend a seminar, we have to ask for permission a thousand times! And, we do that for no other reason but to learn something new in our area, to improve our knowledge.*' (Nurse; Focus group 1)

> *'...Basically, administration wants you to be in your department during the 8-hour shift, even if this would mean that you are playing cards on the computer, instead of allowing you to attend a seminar...'* (Physician B; Focus group 1)

Respondents noted that if a specialism is to be implemented successfully, nursing administration needs to provide nurses with both motives to acquire these qualifications and the opportunity to practise in their selected area.

8.4.5.2 Nursing staff shortages and time constraints

Another obstacle to the implementation of the DSN role in Greece identified in all the focus group sessions was related to the significant shortage of nurses, which resulted in time pressures. This was most notable for nurses qualified at first-level degree, who as respondents noted, would be the future DSNs.

In Greece, there are two levels of basic nursing education. A two-year education programme is provided by hospitals or private nursing schools, and the student is granted the title of assistant nurse at graduation. The four-year education programme leads to a first-level Degree in Nursing. Although there is a wide gap between the curricula of the two-year and the four-year education, all graduates have the same job responsibilities in most hospitals.

Respondents referred to the reluctance of the Ministry of Health to provide funding to employ nurses qualified at degree level, which meant that a high percentage were inevitably employed in the private sector. One physician commented:

> *'...we have to cooperate with unqualified nurses, if you want to call this cooperation, because I would not! I regret I cannot trust a nurse with such a level of education* [two-year education] *and no other further training, to undertake a multifaceted role as that of a DSN, and neither would I recommend her to my patients.'* (Physician B; Focus group 1)

In fact, one 'two-year' nurse reported that she did not have the appropriate knowledge and skills in diabetes, and therefore, could not 'stand by the doctors' in the team and have input into the organisation of the care for patients with diabetes and their families. She said:

> *'I have not been educated for something like this. How can I express my opinion to the doctor when I do not have the knowledge to do this and I am not confident about what I will say?'* (Nurse A; Focus group 5)

8.4.5.3 Medical dominance and the traditional image of the nurse

The final constraint identified by respondents referred to the paternalistic medical system that dominates in the Greek healthcare sector. Most physicians did not agree with the idea of the DSN practising autonomously, namely, without supervision by the medical staff. This was in part attributed to the fact that nurses in Greece have not yet proved that they are able to practise at such an advanced level. Moreover, in many hospitals, the perception relating to nurses' role as 'doctor's handmaidens' dominates. One respondent reported:

> '...*They* [nurses] *give the impression of underestimating their role, bending their head, not having any opinion, and making their role lowly. As result, doctors treat them accordingly.'* (Nurse A; Focus group 3)

Other respondents agreed with the above assertions and noted that many nurses consider working in the field of diabetes care as an easy and convenient option. They are not interested in expanding their role and undertaking further responsibilities. Nurses surmised that undertaking the advanced responsibilities which are currently part of physicians' practice would be a long and difficult process. An additional hindrance to them being able to achieve such an advanced level of practice is the surfeit of physicians: there are twice as many as are currently needed. Moreover, a considerable percentage of patients with diabetes attend physicians' private consultancies for their follow-up care. Therefore, there is a danger that the implementation of the DSN role in the healthcare sector can be perceived by the medical profession as a threat to their territory. As one respondent stated, 'physicians could not afford to lose their clients'.

It was interesting, however, to find that physicians who had previous experience of working with DSNs in other countries strongly supported the implementation of this role in Greece and saw it as a necessity. They did not agree with the opinion of other physicians that DSNs should limit their practice in education activities, but believed that the DSN should be involved in all the advanced activities incorporating the DSN role. One physician commented:

> *'...in Greece there is a wrong mentality regarding the relationship between doctors and nurses, which in my opinion is unacceptable. ...This mentality must change and doctors must accept the DSN as an equal member of the diabetes team if this role is to be successful.'* (Physician A; Focus group 3)

8.4.6 Required qualifications and attributes of the DSN

Respondents were asked to identify the qualifications that they believed a nurse in Greece should acquire in order to become a DSN. All respondents perceived it essential for the nurse to obtain an initial first-level Degree in Nursing; nurses with two-year education should not be considered. Furthermore, respondents stated that the nurse should undertake a minimum of one year's additional postgraduate education to include both theoretical education and clinical attachments. Respondents stressed that the nurses should not be granted the title of DSN based solely on their long-term experience in this field, although a consideration should be given to this factor. They suggested that experienced nurses should also undertake further education and expressed the need for nursing administration to assist nurses in this process.

In addition to formal education, respondents identified a wide range of personal characteristics and attributes necessary for a successful DSN. Such characteristics were disposition, interest, enthusiasm, zeal, 'good spirit and love for patients with diabetes', understanding, 'smiling and having a human approach', patience and perseverance. The importance of personal attributes was particularly highlighted by patients, with one commenting:

'Apart from their scientific competence, I believe that DSNs should have the right disposition to deal with people, to have lots of patience and understanding and put their whole heart into what they do.' (Patient A; Focus group 1)

8.4.7 The pathway to the successful implementation of the DSN role in Greece

Respondents were asked to suggest the pathway which should be followed for the successful implementation of the DSN role in Greece. The initial step would be to prepare nurses through formal education. They suggested that a national educational programme for the speciality should be organised in cooperation with the University of Nursing and selected diabetes centres. However, the most important thing would be for the DSN role to be legally formalised because, as one nurse noted, '…without having that our hands are tied'.

Respondents perceived it necessary that the DSN job description should be agreed jointly by candidate DSNs, nursing administration and physicians. Many respondents stated that it is important for the managers of diabetes centres to have the authority to select and employ their specialist nurses. However, as already noted, the DSN role is unknown in the Greek setting and there is no evidence of its benefits. A number of respondents expressed fears that the Ministry of Health would not provide funding for such a position. One respondent referred to the 'vicious circle' that may occur:

'…the Ministry of Health will not advertise any DSN positions, unless there is evidence that this role can benefit patient care. However, there can be no evidence that this role "works" in the Greek healthcare system, unless it is being implemented and the outcome evaluated' (Nurse B; Focus group 2)

Other respondents suggested that the solution to these problems would be a 'working together' between all health professionals and managers of diabetes centres, and nurses must be initiators of this process. The concluding question asked in the present study was: 'Do you believe that the DSN role can be implemented in Greece in the near future?'. None of the respondents believed that this would happen, in view of the various difficulties that the Greek healthcare system has yet to overcome. An overwhelming response was: 'I do not think so! Perhaps in ten years!' They felt that problems arising from the combination of all the constraints and obstacles reported above cannot be resolved 'from one year to the next'. One respondent reported characteristically:

'I can acquire some specialisation in diabetes and be able to undertake such an advanced role. However, my knowledge and skills will do nothing, unless the whole structure of the healthcare system changes, starting with the Ministry of Health to the way that patients' appointments are arranged in our centre. Then I would be able to apply my skills and improve patient care.' (Nurse A; Focus group 5)

8.5 Discussion

It can be concluded from the results of this study that the DSN role is viewed as 'unreachable' at present in the Greek healthcare system. This role was seen as necessary in the care of people with diabetes, but respondents believed that there are many obstacles preventing its successful implementation.

The exploration of the feasibility of applying the DSN role in Greece was guided by the UK model of the DSN role explored in the previous chapters of this book. Although it is difficult to make direct cross-cultural comparisons between the UK and Greece, it is evident that the successful implementation of the DSN role in the UK was a long and painstaking process and was not achieved from one day to the next. Almost two decades ago, it was stressed that the implementation of this role would be slow and difficult in the first years because of competition for resources and until DSNs had proved their talents and worth (Kinson and Nattrass, 1984). Therefore, it is the author's opinion that with increased efforts from all significant parties, the obstacles to the implementation of the DSN role in Greece can be overcome.

Findings revealed a wide variation in the responsibilities and qualifications of nurses working in the diabetes centres. This is a result of the lack of a standardised job description based on nurses' qualifications and professional experience. As respondents in this study reported, the acquisition of advanced education does not provide them with any professional distinction or promotion in the clinical area. This may be in part due to the fact that the nursing profession, not only in Greece but worldwide, has neither agreed nor clarified that advanced preparation at postgraduate level makes a difference in nursing care delivery (Hamric, 1992).

The results of the present study suggested that nursing in Greece has the ability to prepare advanced practitioners with the appropriate skills to undertake the role of the DSN. It is, therefore, the responsibility of the Ministry of Health and nursing administration to use the knowledge of these nurses appropriately. It is crucial that common objectives are set for nursing practice in general and that of the DSN in particular if the DSN role is to be implemented successfully.

Respondents in the focus groups perceived the implementation of the DSN role in Greece as necessary. The advantages of this role identified by respondents referred to the improvement in patient care, consultation and education, reduction of treatment cost for diabetes, and an increase of the nurse's status and profile in the healthcare service. Similar findings were reported by Richmond (2004) who explored general nurses' perceptions in relation to the recently implemented CNS role in Ireland.

Physicians in the focus groups saw diabetes education as 'time-consuming' for them and preferred the DSN to undertake this role. Nurses, however, did not see this role as simply relieving physicians, but considered themselves to be the most appropriate professionals to undertake diabetes education. Therefore, as the teaching role of the DSN is widely accepted, this may well be an initial step in the implementation of the DSN role in Greece. Nevertheless, future DSNs should aim to expand their role progressively and incorporate all the other components of the DSN role into their practice. Over 20 years ago, Edlund and Hodges (1983: p506) argued that:

> *'...a clear-cut job description, the specialist's title, and the position in the organisational structure must be established prior to the specialist assuming the position. ...The vagueness and lack of specificity regarding role expectations can set the clinical specialist up for failure.'*

As discussed in previous chapters, this assertion was strongly supported by DSNs in the UK. However, in a medically-dominated system, such as that currently existing in Greece, it would be unrealistic to expect the DSN to be able to undertake a multifaceted role from the outset. Kerrison (1990) reported one strategy with which DSNs in the UK expanded their role under a proxy medical model. Physicians 'promoted' their role, as it allowed the delegation of psychosocial work in which nurses claimed greater expertise. By taking on this work, nurses furthered their aspirations for professional status, but did not admit taking over medical work, which in turn avoided overt confrontation with the medical staff, as this would only result in the withdrawal of their support. Were this strategy to be adopted in Greece, it would provide nurses with an opportunity to prove their knowledge and skills not only to other health professionals, but also to patients, and to integrate into the team as an advanced practitioner.

As noted earlier, one of the obstacles to the implementation of the DSN role in Greece is attributed to the medically-dominated healthcare system which often expects the nurse to be 'doctors' handmaidens'. The physician-nurse relationship has been widely explored in the literature (King, 1990; Reigle and Boyle, 2000; Spross, 1989). Brown (1983: p154) stated:

> *'Some physicians and hospital administrators may not be at ease with nurses (or women) who are skilled in presenting their ideas. This changing profile of the female nurse may in some settings produce resistance to the CNS role or to the CNS's ideas.'*

It is assumed that the non-acceptance of the multifaceted role of the DSN in Greece can be attributed to the lack of familiarity with the role. The literature suggests that the CNS, including that of the DSN, developed rapidly in the USA and the UK in response to the shortfall in medical staff. However, findings of the present study revealed a surfeit of physicians in the Greek healthcare setting. This can hinder the acceptance of the DSN role by physicians who may view the DSN as a threat to 'taking over their clients'. Therefore, increased efforts should be made by future DSNs in order to clarify that their role is not aimed at substituting for the role of physicians. Rather these two roles should complement each other in improving standards of care for people with diabetes and their families.

8.6 Strengths, limitations of the study and implications for practice

For the first time, the present study provided the nursing literature with a documentation of the responsibilities and qualifications of nurses working in the diabetes field in Greece. In addition, this was the first step in introducing the DSN role in the Greek health setting. It raised the awareness of health professionals and patients regarding this role by providing evidence from its implementation in the UK. Perceptions of respondents in this study with respect to the benefits and advantages of implementing the DSN role in Greece can be used as evidence to support the need for it in the care of people with diabetes.

The advantages of implementing the DSN role in Greece identified by respondents related to improved patient care and establishment of nurses' status as expert and advanced practitioners. However, the main obstacles to its implementation referred to the status quo of nursing administration, the nursing staff shortages, particularly of appropriately qualified nurses, the medical dominance and the traditional image of the nurse. The identified constraints provide evidence and a basis for the design of strategies to overcome them.

Nursing managers need to understand the complex nature of the role and provide support and career opportunities to future DSNs. Similarly, physicians must be fully informed of its purpose, so that they do not view the DSN as either their assistant or a threat to their professional territory, but as an equal member of the multidisciplinary team. Additionally, future DSNs must make explicit their role expectations and responsibilities to other health professionals in order to assist them to set realistic expectations for this role and avoid its misuse.

Moreover, respondents referred to the necessary qualifications and characteristics of the future DSN. This information can provide useful guidelines in the organisation of the educational curriculum for the preparation of DSNs, should this role be implemented in Greece. Respondents also suggested strategies and pathways for the successful implementation of the DSN role, although they did not see this happening in the near future. These strategies, however, can provide guidelines and 'first-hand evidence' to policy makers in implementing the DSN role in Greece.

The DSN role is a new and almost unknown concept for the Greek setting, and thus it was anticipated that the exploration of its relevance to this setting would be difficult. The seminar presentation to introduce and describe it was found to be significant to the success of this study. However, it was felt that more information needed to be provided to participants in order for them to become familiar with and express their opinions regarding such a complex and multifaceted role as that of the DSN. The fact that many respondents characterised the DSN as something 'unreachable' could, in part, be attributed to their insufficient knowledge of the role.

As the role has not been introduced into this setting, implementation will be difficult. The constraints analysed earlier act as inhibitors to its implementation. Therefore, it is crucial that all significant parties, i.e. government, managers of diabetes centres and diabetes outpatient clinics, nursing administration and health professionals, are informed about and understand the benefits of the DSN role. Evidence of its benefits in other countries should be provided and disseminated through conferences, seminars and publications in both nursing and medical journals. It is important for the policy-makers in the organisation to realise that if the standards and targets set by the St Vincent Declaration (Workshop Report, 1990) are to be achieved, nursing must have a key role in the provision of care. This can only be achieved by introducing advanced nursing roles, such as that of the DSN.

This study elicited data only from the public sector, although the care of a considerable percentage of patients with diabetes in Greece is undertaken in the private sector, which is almost exclusively covered by physicians. It would be useful to explore how the concept of the DSN role is perceived and whether it is acceptable in the private setting.

To conclude, findings from the focus group interviews, as literature suggests, are not replicable and cannot be generalised to the wider population. However, as seven diabetes centres were included in this study, one might expect that this sample is a reasonably accurate reflection of the thirteen centres currently operating around the country.

Nevertheless, it is inappropriate to project findings to the overall diabetes care services provision in Greece. Further studies are recommended to provide a comprehensive exploration of this area and evidence of the need of this role. Further investigation must also be undertaken in order to identify a suitable strategy for the introduction of the DSN role in the Greek healthcare system.

APPENDIX A

THE ROLE OF THE DIABETES SPECIALIST NURSE (DSN) IN THE UK

ORIGINAL QUESTIONNAIRE

SECTION A: PERSONAL CHARACTERISTICS, ATTRIBUTES AND SKILLS

Please indicate your agreement or disagreement with the following statements which express your personal attributes, skills and characteristics as a Diabetes Specialist Nurse. For each of the following, circle a number in the appropriate column on the right.

		Strongly disagree	Disagree	Uncertain	Agree	Strongly agree
1.	I believe I had adequate level of competence in the provision of diabetes care before I entered the DSN post	1	2	3	4	5
2.	I feel I should undertake further education (academic qualification[s]) in order to maintain and/or increase my competence as a DSN	1	2	3	4	5
3.	I consider myself to be a creative person within my role(job)	1	2	3	4	5
4.	I believe I am currently highly competent in the provision of diabetes care	1	2	3	4	5
5.	There is a high degree of flexibility in my role	1	2	3	4	5
6.	I am reluctant to try out new ideas within the context of my role(job)unless I am sure that they will work	1	2	3	4	5
7.	Sometimes I have doubts about my abilities to perform sufficiently my role as a DSN	1	2	3	4	5
8.	Sometimes I feel that my role(job) offers me little motivation or challenge	1	2	3	4	5
9.	I believe I have good communication and interpersonal skills	1	2	3	4	5
10.	I am able to defend and justify the need for change within my practice	1	2	3	4	5
11.	I believe I listen well to concerns of others	1	2	3	4	5
12.	Any ambiguities or constraints in the system within which I work cause me much anxiety and frustration	1	2	3	4	5
13.	I am able to make fast decisions within my practice	1	2	3	4	5
14.	I have difficulties in finding the right solutions to different problems or situations within my practice	1	2	3	4	5
15.	I am familiar with the organisational structure of my work setting and able to identify who has formal and informal power to influence the system	1	2	3	4	5
16.	I have difficulties in negotiating with the administrative authority in favour of improvement in the quality of patient care and/or my working conditions	1	2	3	4	5
17.	I am diligent in my efforts to bring about improvement in my area of practice	1	2	3	4	5

Please go to the next page

SECTION B: WORK SETTING AND ORGANISATIONAL FACTORS

Please indicate your agreement or disagreement with the following statements which represent the work setting and organisational factors that are assumed to influence your role performance as a diabetes specialist nurse. For each of the following, circle a number in the appropriate column on the right.

		Strongly disagree	Disagree	Uncertain	Agree	Strongly agree	Does not apply to my role
1.	My job description states very clearly and precisely what my role tasks and duties include	1	2	3	4	5	6
2.	I currently find that my personal role expectations/goals are incompatible with those of my employing organisation or administrative authority	1	2	3	4	5	6
3	The hospital medical staff are very supportive of my role as a DSN.	1	2	3	4	5	6
4.	I experience difficulties in my professional co-operation with the majority of the community and/or district nurses.	1	2	3	4	5	6
5.	All the members of the healthcare team within which I work are very co-operative and supportive of my role	1	2	3	4	5	6
5.	Hospital nurses frequently ask for my assistance on different issues and problems related to their practice in diabetes care	1	2	3	4	5	6
7.	Most general practitioners are co-operative and supportive of my role	1	2	3	4	5	6
8.	I find that my manager (the person to whom I directly report) does not have a clear understanding of my role as a DSN	1	2	3	4	5	6
9.	My peers/other DSNs provide me with their support and assistance when I have problems or queries related to my practice	1	2	3	4	5	6
10.	The size and/or spread of my current caseload causes me problems in time management and/or performance of my role	1	2	3	4	5	6
11.	My role(job) provides me with professional autonomy and independence.	1	2	3	4	5	6
12.	I am not satisfied with the salary I get from my job	1	2	3	4	5	6
13.	I am provided with sufficient non-clinical material resources by my organisation, such as computer and internet technology, library, etc	1	2	3	4	5	6
14.	I have difficulties in acquiring adequate funding and/or study leave to undertake further academic education related to my area of expertise	1	2	3	4	5	6
15.	I am provided with adequate opportunities and/or funding for outside professional activities (conferences, seminars, study days, etc.)	1	2	3	4	5	6

Please go to the next page

SECTION C(a): DEVELOPMENTAL PHASES OF THE DSN ROLE

The following statements pertain to hypothesised phases (stages) of DSN role development. It is not assumed that you experience all these phases, nor do you necessarily go through them in sequence. In addition, you may feel you are in more than one phase simultaneously or you may repeat phases. Please read the definition of each phase and respond to the questions; I am interested in your professional growth experiences in your current DSN post.

1. How many years have you been in your current DSN post? . . . .

2. Is this your ☐ First ☐ Second, or ☐ Other (please specify.......... DSN post?

3. Orientation phase – characterised by enthusiasm, optimism and anxiety on entry to the DSN post; eager to prove self and make changes that would benefit the organisation and improve quality of care.

a. To what extent have you experienced an **orientation** phase?

Not at all	To a limited extent	To a moderate extent	To a considerable extent	To a great extent
1	2	3	4	5

b. Please describe briefly the reason why you had or did not have this experience. . . . .
. . . .
. . . .
. . . .

4. Frustration phase – characterised by depression and discouragement in the face of slow progress in solving problems due to unrealistic expectations (either self or employer); resistance encountered in the effort to make change. Feels inadequate, overwhelmed, and under pressure to prove worth.

a. To what extent have you experienced a **frustration** phase?

Not at all	To a limited extent	To a moderate extent	To a considerable extent	To a great extent
1	2	3	4	5

b. Please describe briefly the reason why you had or did not have this experience. . . . .
. . . .
. . . .
. . . .

5. Implementation phase – characterised by organisation and reorganisation of role tasks in response to feedback. Returning optimism and enthusiasm. Feelings of being accepted and able to assess situations objectively; implement and balance new sub-roles. Have regained sense of perspective and may focus on specific project(s).

a. To what extent have you experienced an **implementation** phase?

Not at all	To a limited extent	To a moderate extent	To a considerable extent	To a great extent
1	2	3	4	5

b. Please describe briefly the reason why you had or did not have this experience . . . .
. . . .
. . . .
. . . .

Please go to the next page

6. **Integration phase** – characterised by self-confidence, assurance and continuous challenge within role; moderate or great satisfaction with present position; advanced level of practice which reflects wide recognition and influence in area of specialty. Undertakes new projects and expands practice. Congruence between personal and institutional goals/expectations.

a. To what extent have you experienced an **integration** phase?

Not at all	To a limited extent	To a moderate extent	To a considerable extent	To a great extent
1	2	3	4	5

b. Please describe briefly the reason why you had or did not have this experience. . . . .

7. **Frozen phase** – characterised by self-confidence within role and intermediate or advanced level of practice. Conflict between self-expectations and those of national administration of nursing, employing organisation, and/or manager (supervisor). Experiences anger and frustration, and reports being unable to move forward due to forces outside of self.

a. To what extent have you experienced a **frozen** phase?

Not at all	To a limited extent	To a moderate extent	To a considerable extent	To a great extent
1	2	2	4	5

b. Please describe briefly the reason why you had or did not have this experience . . . .

8. **Reorganisation phase** – characterised by self-confidence within role and earlier experiences that represent integration phase. The employing organisation experiences major changes and exerts pressure on the DSN to change his/her role in ways that are incongruent with own concept of role. Experiences stress and conflict in personal goals due to pressure to conform to organisational requirements.

a. To what extent have you experienced a **reorganisation** phase?

Not at all	To a limited extent	To a moderate extent	To a considerable extent	To a great extent
1	2	3	4	5

b. Please describe briefly the reason why you had or did not have this experience . . . .

9. **Complacent phase** – characterised by stability and comfort within role based on the length of experience; variable job satisfaction. Absence of challenge to effect/make change and constructs practice to meet selected, narrowly-focused needs; questionable impact on practice setting/organisation.

a. To what extent have you experienced a **complacent** phase?

Not at all	To a limited extent	To a moderate extent	To a considerable extent	To a great extent
1	2	3	4	5

b. Please describe briefly the reason why you had or did not have this experience. . . . .

Please go to the next page

10. Please indicate the order in which you have experienced these phases by starting with 1 for the first phase you experienced in your current DSN post.

Orientation phase ....
Frustration phase ....
Implementation phase ....
Integration phase ....
Frozen phase ....
Reorganisation phase ....
Complacent phase ....

11. If none of the phases represents your role development experience, please use the space on the back of this page to describe your role development in your current DSN post.

SECTION C(b) : GENERAL ROLE DEVELOPMENT

1. Considering your overall experience as a DSN, what SINGLE factor do you consider as being the most helpful in your role development?

....

2. Considering your overall experience as a DSN, what SINGLE factor do you consider as being the greatest barrier or obstacle in your role development?

....

SECTION D(a): ROLE PERFORMANCE OF THE DSN: ROLE COMPONENTS

Within the past year or so, indicate by circling a number in the appropriate column on the right how often you perform each activity that best describes your role as a diabetes specialist nurse.

		Not at all	Rarely	Occasionally	Frequently	Very frequently
	Expert practitioner, Care giver					
1	Collaborate with team members and other healthcare staff in assessing, planning, implementing, and evaluating comprehensive diabetes care	1	2	3	4	5
2	Adminster routine direct patient care in the field of diabetes	1	2	3	4	5
3	Assess and adjust insulin dosages as required	1	2	3	4	5
4	Adjust oral hypoglycaemic drugs	1	2	3	4	5
5	Prescribe diabetes-related medications	1	2	3	4	5
6	Order laboratory tests and diagnostic procedures	1	2	3	4	5
7	Provide specialised direct care requiring advanced skills and knowledge to patients with complex physical problems and their families/carers	1	2	3	4	5
8	Carry a caseload of patients with diabetes and establish long and short-term goals for care of individual patients	1	2	3	4	5
9	Participate in interdisciplinary patient care conferences	1	2	3	4	5
10	Provide advice and support to patients and/or their families via telephone	1	2	3	4	5

Please go to the next page

		Not at all	Rarely	Occasionally	Frequently	Very frequently
11	Provide an out-of-hours help-line for emergency cases	1	2	3	4	5
12	Carry out home visits to maintain follow-up in patient care	1	2	3	4	5
13	Act as a role model for staff and students when performing care	1	2	3	4	5
14	Act as a patient advocate in clinical practice	1	2	3	4	5
	Educator					
15	Co-ordinate and/or participate in the education and training of nursing staff	1	2	3	4	5
16	Provide education to medical staff	1	2	3	4	5
17	Contribute to the educational and professional development of nursing and/or other healthcare students	1	2	3	4	5
18	Develop/participate in the development, implementation, and/or evaluation of educational resources and materials that facilitate diabetes education	1	2	3	4	5
19	Plan, initiate and evaluate individual patient teaching programmes	1	2	3	4	5
20	Plan, implement, and evaluate group teaching of patients and their families	1	2	3	4	5
21	Co-ordinate and/or participate in community and public educational and informational programmes	1	2	3	4	5
22	Take part in the delivery of formal academic education in diabetes	1	2	3	4	5
23	Organise, in collaboration with other members of the healthcare team, seminars on diabetes and workshops for healthcare professionals	1	2	3	4	5
24	Provide diabetes education to people who are in contact with the person with diabetes, such as school teachers, employers, friends, etc	1	2	3	4	5
	Consultant, Advisor					
25	Consult with nurse managers/ward sisters to identify clinical activities that facilitate the professional growth of the nursing staff	1	2	3	4	5
26	Provide leadership in the assessment, development, and/or implementation of policies, protocols, procedures, and care pathways in my area of practice	1	2	3	4	5
27	Participate in setting and/or implementing standards and targets of diabetes in my area of practice and/or health board (district)	1	2	3	4	5
28	Participate in setting standards of diabetes care at a national level	1	2	3	4	5
29	Facilitate the organisation of patient support groups in my area of practice or health board/trust/district	1	2	3	4	5
30	Act as a resource person for staff and students in the area of diabetes care	1	2	3	4	5
31	Function on an 'on-call' basis for nursing and/or other staff who need assistance in solving complex problems related to diabetes care	1	2	3	4	5
32	Provide answers to clinical problems identified by healthcare personnel or try/know where to find the answers when not available	1	2	3	4	5
33	Help patients with diabetes and their families/carers to cope with the immediate crisis of diagnosis and long-term adjustments in life style	1	2	3	4	5
	Researcher					
34	Identify nursing care problems and develop relevant questions appropriate for systematic study	1	2	3	4	5
35	Conduct research-related diabetes and/or other areas of nursing practice	1	2	3	4	5
36	Communicate own research findings through presentations or publications.	1	2	3	4	5
37	Disseminate own and/or other research findings to staff and suggest appropriate means of implementing these in practice	1	2	3	4	5

Please go to the next page

		Not at all	Rarely	Occasionally	Frequently	Very frequently
38	Participate in (a) nursing research committee(s)	1	2	3	4	5
39	Collaborate with other healthcare professionals in research	1	2	3	4	5
40	Participate in product evaluation	1	2	3	4	5
41	Develop proposals for funding nursing research	1	2	3	4	5
42	Contribute to the nursing literature through publications	1	2	3	4	5
43	Act as a preceptor and resource for staff/students conducting research.	1	2	3	4	5
44	Develop and conduct patient outcome evaluations.	1	2	3	4	5
	Manager, Administrator					
45	Participate in financial and budget planning for diabetes specialty areas	1	2	3	4	5
46	Represent nursing administration in the review of policies and procedures of departmental and/or institutional committees	1	2	3	4	5
47	Perform or provide input into staff evaluations	1	2	3	4	5
48	Participate in decisions regarding employment of nursing personnel	1	2	3	4	5
49	Participate in identifying gaps in the diabetes care services.	1	2	3	4	5
	Collaborator, Communicator, Liaison					
50	Communicate and interpret nursing assessment of people with diabetes to medical staff and other relevant health personnel	1	2	3	4	5
51	Co-ordinate and facilitate transfer or discharge planning between different care settings (primary-secondary-tertiary care) and/or departments	1	2	3	4	5
52	Initiate, direct, and/or facilitate patient referrals to appropriate healthcare professionals and/or community resources/agencies.	1	2	3	4	5
53	Utilise and co-ordinate the varied resources and facilities for diabetes care in my area of practice.	1	2	3	4	5
	Change agent, Innovator					
54	Implement in practice recent innovations and research findings related to diabetes care and evaluate their impact on the quality of care	1	2	3	4	5
55	Implement and evaluate appropriate nursing models in the care of people with diabetes and their families/carers	1	2	3	4	5
56	Identify, implement, and evaluate in collaboration with healthcare staff new ways of improving diabetes care	1	2	3	4	5
57	Design presentations for the administrative authority, outlining needs for change and feasible steps for realising the goals	1	2	3	4	5
58	Continuously monitor and assess changing needs of diabetes care, and institute/facilitate appropriate change	1	2	3	4	5

Please go to the next page

SECTION D(b):

Please indicate (approximately) the **percentages** of your total work time that you recently spent in each of the following role components and activities. If the components sometimes overlap, divide the time between them so that the total working time equals 100%.

	Role components	Time allotted
1.	Expert practitioner/Care giver	--------------%
2.	Educator	--------------%
3.	Consultant/Advisor.	--------------%
4.	Researcher	--------------%
5.	Manager/Administrator	--------------%
6.	Miscellaneous (travelling, lunch, etc.)	--------------% (Should total 100%)

SECTION E: DEMOGRAPHIC CHARACTERISTICS, PRACTICE IN CURRENT POST, EDUCATIONAL (ACADEMIC) QUALIFICATIONS

1. In which of the following NHS Executive Regions do you work?

   [1] Eastern [2] London [3] North West [4] Scotland [5] Northern & Yorkshire

   [6] South East [7] South West [8] Trent [9] Wales [10] West Midlands

2. What of the following qualification(s) do you have?

   O RGN O RSCN O DN O RHV

3. What is your current grade?

   O E O F O G O H O I O Other (please specify)....

4. What is your employment status as DSN?

   O Full-time O Part-time

5. Which of the following best describes your work setting?

   O Hospital based O Community based

   O Between hospital and community O Other (please specify) ....

6. Do you work with: O Children O Adults or O Both?

7. What is the size of your diabetes caseload at the moment? . . . .

8. What is the district population of the area that you cover in your practice? . . . .

9. How many DSNs are employed in your practice setting or institution? . . . .

10. Which of the following statements best describes your placement in the organisational chart?

    O I have administrative authority in the management of human and/or financial resources in my area of practice (line position)

    O I have no direct responsibility in the management of service and its resources; I often act as consultant or advisor regarding the organisation of diabetes care services (staff position)

    O Other (please specify) . . . .

11. Do you have a peer support group with other DSNs?

    O Yes ———▶ **If yes**, please indicate the approximate interval of time between meetings . . . .
    O No . . . .

12. What is the highest educational (academic) qualification you have earned in nursing?

    O Diploma O Master's Degree

    O Degree O Doctorate

    O Postgraduate diploma O Others (please specify)..............................

Please go to the next page

13. Have you undergone/are you presently undergoing further education or training to prepare you specifically for your role as a diabetes specialist nurse?

O Yes ——▶ **If yes**, please tick the course(s) or other training that you have undertaken/are undertaking related to diabetes nursing specialty

O No

[1] National Board Courses-928

[2] Other National Board Course(s)

[3] Specialist UKCC recordable diabetes qualification

[4] Accredited short course(s) in diabetes

[5] Non-accredited short course(s) in diabetes

[6] BSc (Hons) in Specialist Practice

[7] Diploma (please specify) . . . .

[8] Graduate Certificate (please specify) . . . .

[9] Postgraduate Diploma (please specify). . . . .

[10] Master's Degree (please specify). . . . .

[11] Other (please specify) . . . .

14. Have you undertaken/are you presently undertaking any educational (academic) qualification which is not relevant to diabetes but has contributed or you believe it will contribute to the integration of your role as a DSN?

O Yes ——▶ **If yes**, please specify the type of education and the reason why it has contributed/you believe it will contribute to the integration of your role . . . .

O No

. . . .

. . . .

. . . .

15. How satisfied are you with your current position as a DSN?

O Very dissatisfied

O Moderately dissatisfied

O Partly dissatisfied-partly satisfied

O Moderately satisfied

O Very satisfied

I would like to express my sincere appreciation and gratitude for your time and support with this project. Please use the space on the back of this page should you wish to comment on any issues raised in this questionnaire.

Please return survey to: ....

....

....

APPENDIX B

THE ROLE OF THE DIABETES SPECIALIST NURSE (DSN) IN THE UK

Validated Questionnaire based on the Role Theory Framework

SECTION A: PERSONAL CHARACTERISTICS, ATTRIBUTES, AND SKILLS

Please indicate your agreement or disagreement with the following statements which express your personal attributes, skills and characteristics as a diabetes specialist nurse. For each of the following, circle a number in the appropriate column on the right.

	Strongly disagree	Disagree	Uncertain	Agree	Strongly agree
Competence Within Role					
I believe I am currently highly competent in the provision of diabetes care	1	2	3	4	5
I am able to defend and justify the need for change within my practice	1	2	3	4	5
There is a high degree of flexibility in my role	1	2	3	4	5
I am able to make fast decisions within my practice	1	2	3	4	5
I have difficulties in finding the right solutions to different problems or situations within my practice	1	2	3	4	5
I am reluctant to try out new ideas within the context of my role(job) unless I am sure that they will work	1	2	3	4	5
Sometimes I have doubts about my abilities to perform sufficiently my role as a DSN	1	2	3	4	5
Organisational Issues					
I have difficulties in negotiating with the administrative authority in favour of improvement in the quality of patient care and/or my working conditions	1	2	3	4	5
I am familiar with the organisational structure of my work setting and able to identify who has formal and informal power to influence the system	1	2	3	4	5
Any ambiguities or constraints in the system within which I work cause me much anxiety and frustration	1	2	3	4	5
Sometimes I feel that my role(job) offers me little motivation or challenge	1	2	3	4	5
Personal Attributes					
I believe I listen well to concerns of others	1	2	3	4	5
I believe I have good communication and interpersonal skills	1	2	3	4	5
I am diligent in my efforts to bring about improvement in my area of practice	1	2	3	4	5
I consider myself to be a creative person within my role(job)	1	2	3	4	5

Please go to the next page

SECTION B: WORK SETTING AND ORGANISATIONAL FACTORS

Please indicate your agreement or disagreement with the following statements which represent the work setting and organisational factors that are assumed to influence your role performance as a Diabetes Specialist Nurse. For each of the following, circle a number in the appropriate column on the right.

	Strongly disagree	Disagree	Uncertain	Agree	Strongly agree	Does not apply to my role
Collaborative Working						
All the members of the healthcare team within which I work are very co-operative and supportive of my role	1	2	3	4	5	6
The hospital medical staff are very supportive of my role as a DSN	1	2	3	4	5	6
My role(job) provides me with professional autonomy and independence	1	2	3	4	5	6
Hospital nurses frequently ask for my assistance on different issues and problems related to their practice in diabetes care	1	2	3	4	5	6
Most general practitioners are co-operative and supportive of my role	1	2	3	4	5	6
I experience difficulties in my professional co-operation with the majority of the community and/or district nurses	1	2	3	4	5	6
My peers/other DSNs provide me with their support and assistance when I have problems or queries related to my practice	1	2	3	4	5	6
Role Expectations						
I currently find that my personal role expectations/goals are incompatible with those of my employing organisation or administrative authority	1	2	3	4	5	6
My job description states very clearly and precisely what my role tasks and duties include	1	2	3	4	5	6
I find that my manager (the person to whom I directly report) does not have a clear understanding of my role as a DSN	1	2	3	4	5	6
The size and/or spread of my current caseload causes me problems in time management and/or performance of my role	1	2	3	4	5	6
I am not satisfied with the salary I get from my job	1	2	3	4	5	6
Resources						
I am provided with adequate opportunities and/or funding for outside professional activities (conferences, seminars, study days, etc.)	1	2	3	4	5	6
I have difficulties in acquiring adequate funding and/or study leave to undertake further academic education related to my area of expertise	1	2	3	4	5	6
I am provided with sufficient non-clinical material resources by my organisation, such as computer and internet technology, library, etc	1	2	3	4	5	6

Please go to the next page

SECTION C (a): DEVELOPMENTAL PHASES OF THE DSN ROLE

The following statements pertain to hypothesised phases (stages) of DSN role development. It is not assumed that you experience all these phases, nor do you necessarily go through them in sequence. In addition, you may feel you are in more than one phase simultaneously or you may repeat phases. Please read the definition of each phase and respond to the questions; I am interested in your professional growth experiences in your current DSN post.

1. How many years have you been in your current DSN post? ....

2. Is this your ☐ First ☐ Second, or ☐ Other (please specify)........... DSN post?

3. Orientation phase – characterised by enthusiasm, optimism and anxiety on entry to the DSN post; eager to prove self and make changes that would benefit the organisation and improve quality of care.

a. To what extent have you experienced an **orientation** phase?

Not at all	To a limited extent	To a moderate extent	To a considerable extent	To a great extent
1	2	3	4	5

b. Please describe briefly the reason why you had or did not have this experience.................................
....
....
....

4. Frustration phase – characterised by depression and discouragement in the face of slow progress in solving problems due to unrealistic expectations (either self or employer); resistance encountered in the effort to make change. Feels inadequate, overwhelmed, and under pressure to prove worth.

a. To what extent have you experienced a **frustration** phase?

Not at all	To a limited extent	To a moderate extent	To a considerable extent	To a great extent
1	2	3	4	5

b. Please describe briefly the reason why you had or did not have this experience.................................
....
....
....

5. Implementation phase – characterised by organisation and reorganisation of role tasks in response to feedback. Returning optimism and enthusiasm. Feelings of being accepted and able to assess situations objectively; implement and balance new sub-roles. Have regained sense of perspective and may focus on specific project(s).

a. To what extent have you experienced an **implementation** phase?

Not at all	To a limited extent	To a moderate extent	To a considerable extent	To a great extent
1	2	3	4	5

b. Please describe briefly the reason why you had or did not have this experience ....
....
....
....

Please go to the next page

6. **Integration phase** – characterised by self-confidence, assurance and continuous challenge within role; moderate or great satisfaction with present position; advanced level of practice which reflects wide recognition and influence in area of specialty. Undertakes new projects and expands practice. Congruence between personal and institutional goals/expectations.

a. To what extent have you experienced an **integration** phase?

Not at all	To a limited extent	To a moderate extent	To a considerable extent	To a great extent
1	2	3	4	5

b. Please describe briefly the reason why you had or did not have this experience. . . . .

. . . .

. . . .

. . . .

7. **Frozen phase** – characterised by self-confidence within role and intermediate or advanced level of practice. Conflict between self-expectations and those of national administration of nursing, employing organisation, and/or manager (supervisor). Experiences anger and frustration, and reports being unable to move forward due to forces outside of self.

a. To what extent have you experienced a **frozen** phase?

Not at all	To a limited extent	To a moderate extent	To a considerable extent	To a great extent
1	2	2	4	5

b. Please describe briefly the reason why you had or did not have this experience . . . .

. . . .

. . . .

. . . .

8. **Reorganisation phase** – characterised by self-confidence within role and earlier experiences that represent integration phase. The employing organisation experiences major changes and exerts pressure on the DSN to change his/her role in ways that are incongruent with own concept of role. Experiences stress and conflict in personal goals due to pressure to conform to organisational requirements.

a. To what extent have you experienced a **reorganisation** phase?

Not at all	To a limited extent	To a moderate extent	To a considerable extent	To a great extent
1	2	3	4	5

b. Please describe briefly the reason why you had or did not have this experience . . . .

. . . .

. . . .

. . . .

9. **Complacent phase** – characterised by stability and comfort within role based on the length of experience; variable job satisfaction. Absence of challenge to effect/make change and constructs practice to meet selected, narrowly-focused needs; questionable impact on practice setting/organisation.

a. To what extent have you experienced a **complacent** phase?

Not at all	To a limited extent	To a moderate extent	To a considerable extent	To a great extent
1	2	3	4	5

b. Please describe briefly the reason why you had or did not have this experience. . . . .

. . . .

. . . .

. . . .

Please go to the next page

10. Transition phase – characterized by enthusiasm and eagerness in bringing about improvement. Self-confidence, competence and advanced level of practice within role. Previous expertise are recognised by team members in the new setting. Feelings of anxiety are related to orientation into a new work setting rather than to the role-related knowledge base.

c. To what extent have you experienced a **orientation** phase?

Not at all	To a limited extent	To a moderate extent	To a considerable extent	To a great extent
1	2	3	4	5

d. Please describe briefly the reason why you had or did not have this experience.......................................

....

....

....

11. Please indicate the order in which you have experienced these phases by starting with **1** for the first phase you experienced in your current DSN post.

Orientation phase ________ Frustration phase ________

Implementation phase ________ Integration phase ________

Frozen phase ________ Reorganisation phase ________

Complacent phase ________ Transition phase ________

12. If none of the phases represents your role development experience, please use the space on the back of this page to describe your role development in your current DSN post.

SECTION C (b): GENERAL ROLE DEVELOPMENT

1 Considering your overall experience as a DSN, what SINGLE factor do you consider as being the most helpful in your role development?

....

2. Considering your overall experience as a DSN, what SINGLE factor do you consider as being the greatest barrier or obstacle in your role development?

....

Please go to the next page

SECTION D(a): ROLE PERFORMANCE OF THE DSN: ROLE COMPONENTS

Within the past year or so, indicate by circling a number in the appropriate column on the right how often you perform each activity that best describes your role as a diabetes specialist nurse.

	Not at all	Rarely	Occasionally	Frequently	Very frequently
1: Expert practitioner, Care giver					
Direct Care					
Administer routine direct patient care in the field of diabetes	1	2	3	4	5
Provide advice and support to patients and/or their families via telephone	1	2	3	4	5
Carry a caseload of patients with diabetes and establish long and short-term goals for care of individual patients	1	2	3	4	5
Assess and adjust insulin dosages as required	1	2	3	4	5
Liaison and Indirect Care					
Act as a patient advocate in clinical practice	1	2	3	4	5
Act as a role model for staff and students when performing care	1	2	3	4	5
Carry out home visits to maintain follow-up in patient care	1	2	3	4	5
Provide an out-of-hours help-line for emergency cases	1	2	3	4	5
Collaborate with team members and other healthcare staff in assessing, planning, implementing, and evaluating comprehensive diabetes care	1	2	3	4	5
Advanced Specialised Care					
Adjust oral hypoglycaemic drugs	1	2	3	4	5
Order laboratory tests and diagnostic procedures	1	2	3	4	5
Provide specialised direct care requiring advanced skills and knowledge to patients with complex physical problems and their families/carers	1	2	3	4	5
Prescribe diabetes-related medications	1	2	3	4	5
2: Educator					
Educating Health Staff					
Co-ordinate and/or participate in the education and training of nursing staff	1	2	3	4	5
Take part in the delivery of formal academic education in diabetes	1	2	3	4	5
Organise, in collaboration with other members of the healthcare team, seminars on diabetes and workshops for healthcare professionals	1	2	3	4	5
Contribute to the educational and professional development of nursing and/or other healthcare students	1	2	3	4	5
Provide education to medical staff	1	2	3	4	5
Educating Patients, Families and Public					
Develop/participate in the development, implementation, and/or evaluation of educational resources and materials that facilitate diabetes education	1	2	3	4	5
Plan, initiate and evaluate individual patient teaching programmes	1	2	3	4	5
Plan, implement, and evaluate group teaching of patients and their families	1	2	3	4	5
Provide diabetes education to people who are in contact with the person with diabetes, such as school teachers, employers, friends, etc	1	2	3	4	5
Co-ordinate and/or participate in community and public educational and informational programmes	1	2	3	4	5

Please go to the next page

	Not at all	Rarely	Occasionally	Frequently	Very frequently
3: Consultant, Advisor					
Consultation regarding the Organisation of Care					
Provide leadership in the assessment, development, and/or implementation of policies, protocols, procedures, and care pathways in my area of practice	1	2	3	4	5
Participate in setting and/or implementing standards and targets of diabetes in my area of practice and/or health board (district)	1	2	3	4	5
Consult with nurse managers/ward sisters to identify clinical activities that facilitate the professional growth of the nursing staff	1	2	3	4	5
Participate in setting standards of diabetes care at a national level	1	2	3	4	5
Facilitate the organisation of patient support groups in my area of practice or health board/trust/district	1	2	3	4	5
Provide answers to clinical problems identified by healthcare personnel or try/know where to find the answers when not available	1	2	3	4	5
Help patients with diabetes and their families/carers to cope with the immediate crisis of diagnosis and long-term adjustments in life style	1	2	3	4	5
Act as a resource person for staff and students in the area of diabetes care	1	2	3	4	5
Function on an 'on-call' basis for nursing and/or other staff who need assistance in solving complex problems related to diabetes care	1	2	3	4	5
4: Researcher					
Communicate own research findings through presentations or publications	1	2	3	4	5
Conduct research-related diabetes and/or other areas of nursing practice	1	2	3	4	5
Disseminate own and/or other research findings to staff and suggest appropriate means of implementing these in practice	1	2	3	4	5
Identify nursing care problems and develop relevant questions appropriate for systematic study	1	2	3	4	5
Develop and conduct patient outcome evaluations	1	2	3	4	5
Collaborate with other healthcare professionals in research	1	2	3	4	5
Develop proposals for funding nursing research	1	2	3	4	5
Act as a preceptor and resource for staff/students conducting research	1	2	3	4	5
Participate in product evaluation	1	2	3	4	5
Participate in (a) nursing research committee(s)	1	2	3	4	5
Contribute to the nursing literature through publications	1	2	3	4	5
5: Manager, Administrator					
Perform or provide input into staff evaluations	1	2	3	4	5
Represent nursing administration in the review of policies and procedures of departmental and/or institutional committees	1	2	3	4	5
Participate in decisions regarding employment of nursing personnel	1	2	3	4	5
Participate in financial and budget planning for diabetes specialty areas	1	2	3	4	5
Participate in identifying gaps in the diabetes care services	1	2	3	4	5

Please go to the next page

	Not at all	Rarely	Occasionally	Frequently	Very frequently
6: Collaborator, Communicator					
Initiate, direct, and/or facilitate patient referrals to appropriate healthcare professionals and/or community resources/agencies.	1	2	3	4	5
Utilise and co-ordinate the varied resources and facilities for diabetes care in my area of practice.	1	2	3	4	5
Co-ordinate and facilitate transfer or discharge planning between different care settings (primary-secondary-tertiary care) and/or departments.	1	2	3	4	5
Communicate and interpret nursing assessment of people with diabetes to medical staff and other relevant health personnel	1	2	3	4	5
7: Change agent, Innovator					
Identify, implement, and evaluate in collaboration with healthcare staff new ways of improving diabetes care	1	2	3	4	5
Implement in practice recent innovations and research findings related to diabetes care and evaluate their impact on the quality of care	1	2	3	4	5
Implement and evaluate appropriate nursing models in the care of people with diabetes and their families/carers	1	2	3	4	5
Continuously monitor and assess changing needs of diabetes care, and institute/facilitate appropriate change.	1	2	3	4	5
Design presentations for the administrative authority, outlining needs for change and feasible steps for realising the goals	1	2	3	4	5

SECTION D(b)

Please indicate (approximately) the **percentages** of your total work time that you recently spent in each of the following role components and activities. If the components sometimes overlap, divide the time between them so that the total working time equals 100%.

	Role components	Time allotted
1.	Expert practitioner/Care giver	--------------%
2.	Educator	--------------%
3.	Consultant/Advisor.	--------------%
4.	Researcher	--------------%
5.	Manager/Administrator	--------------%
6.	Miscellaneous (travelling, lunch, etc.)	--------------% (Should total 100%)

Please go to the next page

SECTION E: DEMOGRAPHIC CHARACTERISTICS, PRACTICE IN CURRENT POST, EDUCATIONAL (ACADEMIC) QUALIFICATIONS

1. In which of the following NHS Executive Regions do you work?

   [1] Eastern [2] London [3] North West [4] Scotland [5] Northern & Yorkshire

   [6] South East [7] South West [8] Trent [9] Wales [10] West Midlands

2. What of the following qualification(s) do you have?

   O RGN O RSCN O DN O RHV

3. What is your current grade?

   O E O F O G O H O I O Other (please specify)....

4. What is your employment status as DSN?

   O Full-time O Part-time

5. Which of the following best describes your work setting?

   O Hospital based O Community based

   O Between hospital and community O Other (please specify) ....

6. Do you work with: O Children O Adults or O Both?

7. What is the size of your diabetes caseload at the moment? ....

8. What is the district population of the area that you cover in your practice? ....

9. How many DSNs are employed in your practice setting or institution? ....

10. Which of the following statements best describes your placement in the organisational chart?

    O I have administrative authority in the management of human and/or financial resources in my area of practice (line position)

    O I have no direct responsibility in the management of service and its resources; I often act as consultant or advisor regarding the organisation of diabetes care services (staff position)

    O Other (please specify)...

11. Do you have a peer support group with other DSNs?

    O Yes ———▶ **If yes,** please indicate the approximate interval of time between meetings ....
    O No ....

12. What is the highest educational (academic) qualification you have earned in nursing?

    O Diploma O Master's Degree

    O Degree O Doctorate

    O Postgraduate diploma O Others (please specify)..............................

Please go to the next page

13. Have you undergone/are you presently undergoing further education or training to prepare you <u>specifically</u> for your role as a diabetes specialist nurse?

O Yes ——▶ **If yes**, please tick the course(s) or other training that you have undertaken/are undertaking related to diabetes nursing specialty

O No

[1] National Board Courses-928

[2] Other National Board Course(s)

[3] Specialist UKCC recordable diabetes qualification

[4] Accredited short course(s) in diabetes

[5] Non-accredited short course(s) in diabetes

[6] BSc (Hons) in Specialist Practice

[7] Diploma (please specify). . . . .

[8] Graduate Certificate (please specify) . . . .

[9] Postgraduate Diploma (please specify). . . . .

[10] Master's Degree (please specify). . . . .

[11] Other (please specify) . . . .

14. Have you undertaken/are you presently undertaking any educational (academic) qualification which is <u>not relevant to diabetes</u> but has contributed or you believe it will contribute to the integration of your role as a DSN?

❍ Yes ——▶ **If yes**, please specify the type of education and the reason why it has contributed/you believe it will contribute to the integration of your role . . . .

❍ No

. . . .

. . . .

. . . .

15. How satisfied are you with your current position as a DSN?

❍ Very dissatisfied

❍ Moderately dissatisfied

❍ Partly dissatisfied-partly satisfied

❍ Moderately satisfied

❍ Very satisfied

I would like to express my sincere appreciation and gratitude for your time and support with this project. Please use the space on the back of this page should you wish to comment on any issues raised in this questionnaire.

Please return survey to: ....

....

....

REFERENCES

Aikin JL, Taggart JR, Tripoli CA (1993) Evaluation and time documentation for the clinical nurse specialist. *Clin Nurse Spec* **7**(1): 33–38

Aitkin TJ, VanArsdale SK, Barry LA (1990) Strategies for practice as a clinical nurse specialist in a small setting. *Clin Nurse Specialist* **4**: 28–32

Alderton J, Freeman M, Miller C (1997). The pivotal role of the nurse in the diabetes team. *J Diabetes Nurs* **1**(4): 118–20

Allen VL, van de Vliert E (1984) A role theoretical perspective on transitional processes. In: Allen VL, van de Vliert E, eds. *Role Transitions: Explorations and Explanations*. Plenum Press, New York: 3–18

Al-Zaru IM (2001) The Jordanian nurses' role as patient educators in acute care settings in the state sector: factors influencing role development. Unpublished PhD Thesis, University of Ulster, Northern Ireland

Ambutas S (1991) Role of the clinical nurse specialist in open heart surgery. *Nurs Manage* **22**: 64A–64D

American Nurses Association (1986) Clinical nurse specialists: distribution and utilisation. Cited in: Sparacino PSA, Cooper DM, Minarik PA (1990) *The Clinical Nurse Specialist: Implementation and Impact*. Appleton and Lange, Norwalk: 54

American Nurses Association (1984) *Issues in Professional Nursing 2: Specialisation in Nursing Practice*. American Nurses Association, Kansas City

American Nurses Association (1980) Nursing: a social policy statement. Cited in: Keeling AW, Bigbee JL (2005). The history of advanced practice nursing in the United States. In: Hamric AB, Spross JA, Hanson CM, eds. *Advanced Practice Nursing: An Integrative Approach*, 3rd edn. Elsevier Saunders, St Louis: 3–45

Anfield J (1998) The Northampton story: DSNs under threat. *J Diabetes Nurs* **2**(1): 4–5

Arber S (1993) Designing samples. In: Gilbert N, ed. *Researching Social Life*. Sage Publications, London: 68–92

Arford PH, Olson M (1988) A structural perspective of nurse manager and clinical nurse specialist collaboration. *Clin Nurse Spec* **2**(3): 119–26

Artinian BM (1982) Conceptual mapping: development of the strategy. *W J Nurs Res* **4**(4): 379–93

Baker PO (1987) Model activities for clinical nurse specialist's role development. *Clin Nurse Spec* **1**(3): 119–23.

Baker V (1979) Retrospective explorations in role development. In: Padilla GV, ed. *The Clinical Nurse Specialist and Improvement of Nursing Practice*. Nursing Resources,Wakefield, MA: 56–63

Bandura A (1977) *Social Learning Theory*. Prentice-Hall, Englewood Cliffs

Banton M (1965) *Roles: An Introduction to the Study of Social Relations*. Tavistock, London

Barron AM (1989) The CNS as consultant. In: Hamric AB, Spross JA, eds. *The Clinical Nurse Specialist in Theory and Practice*, 2nd edn. WB Saunders, Philadelphia: 125–45

Bartsokas CS (1999) The Greek contribution to diabetes research. *Diabetes Metab Res Rev* **15**: 362–72

Beaudry M, Vandenbosch T, Anderson J (1996) Research utilisation: once a day temperatures for afebrile patients. *Clin Nurse Spec* **10**: 21–24

Beecroft PC (2001). Mentors and mentoring: editorial. *Clin Nurse Spec* **15**(3): 89

Beecroft PC, Papenhausen JL (1989) Who is a clinical nurse specialist? *Clin Nurse Spec* **3**(3): 103–104

Beecroft PC, Papenhausen JL (1985) Clinical nurse specialist survey. Unpublished research. Cited in: Topham DL (1987) Role theory in relation to roles of the clinical nurse specialist. *Clin Nurse Spec* **1**(2): 81–84

Benner P (2001) *From Novice to Expert: Excellence and Power in Clinical Nursing Practice*, Commemorative Edition. Prentice Hall Health, Upper Saddle River, New Jersey.

Berger AM, Eilers JG, Heermann JA, Warren JJ, Franco T, Triolo PM (1999) State-of-the-art patient care: the impact of doctorally prepared clinical nurses. *Clin Nurse Spec* **13**(5): 259–66

Biddle BJ (1986) Recent developments in role theory. *Ann Rev Sociol* **12**: 67–92

Biddle BJ (1979) *Role Theory: Expectations, Identities and Behaviours*. Academic Press, New York

Bigbee JL, Amidi-Nouri A (2000) History and evolution of advanced nursing practice. In: Hamric AB, Spross JA, Hanson CM, eds. *Advanced Nursing Practice: An Integrative Approach*, 2nd edn. WB Saunders, Philadelphia: 3–32

Blumer H (1969) *Symbolic Interactionism: Perspective and Method*. University of California Press, Berkeley

Boucher RJ, Bruce SJ (1972) Similarities and differences in perceptions of the role of the clinical specialist: volume I. Valuations of functions of the role of the clinical nursing specialist: volume II. *American Nurse Association Eighth Research Conference*, 163–168

Bousfield C (1997) A phenomenological investigation into the role of the clinical nurse specialist. *J Adv Nurs* **25**: 245–56

Bowman G, Thompson D (1990) When is a specialist not a specialist? *Nurs Times* **86**(8): 48

Boyd NJ, Stasiowski SA, Catoe PT, *et al* (1991) The merit and significance of clinical nurse specialist. *J Nurs Admin* **21**: 35–43

Brake J (1997) Advantages and disadvantages of nurse prescribing. *J Diabetes Nurs* **1**(4): 113–17

Brim OG, jr (1966) Socialisation through the life cycle. In: Brim jr OG, Wheeler S, eds. *Socialisation after Childhood: Two Essays*. Wiley, New York: 1–50

Brim OG, jr (1960) Personality development as role-learning. In: Iscoe I, Stevenson HW, Jones HE, eds. *Personality Development in Children*. University of Texas Press, Austin: 127–59

Brink PJ, Wood MJ (1994) *Basic Steps in Planning Research: From Question to Proposal*, 4th edn. Jones and Bartlett, Boston

British Diabetic Association (1993) *Directory of Diabetes Specialist Nurses*. Diabetes UK, London

Brown SJ (1989) Supportive supervision of the CNS. In: Hamric AB, Spross JA, eds. *The Clinical Nurse Specialist in Theory and Practice*, 2nd edn. WB Saunders, Philadelphia: 285–98

Brown SJ (1983) Administrative support. In: Hamric AB, Spross J, eds. *The Clinical Nurse Specialist in Theory and Practice*. Grune and Stratton, Orlando: 149–70

Brykczynski KA (2005) Role development of the advanced practice nurse. In: Hamric AB, Spross JA, Hanson CM, eds. *Advanced Practice Nursing: An Integrative Approach*, 3rd edn. Elsevier Saunders, Philadelphia: 109–42

Brykczynski KA (2000) Role development of the advanced practice nurse. In: Hamric AB, Spross JA Hanson CM, eds. *Advanced Nursing Practice: An Integrative Approach*, 2nd edn. WB Saunders, Philadelphia: 107–35

Burge S, Crigler S, Hurt L, Kelly G, Sanborn C (1989) Clinical nurse specialist role development: quantifying actual practice over three years. *Clin Nurse Spec* **3**(1): 33–36

Burns N, Grove SK (1997) *The Practice of Nursing Research: Conduct, Critique and Utilisation*, 3rd edn. WB Saunders, Philadelphia

Calkin JD (1988) The effects of organisational structure on role behaviour. In: Hardy ME, Conway ME, eds. *Role Theory: Perspectives for Health Professionals*, 2nd edn. Appleton and Lange, Norwalk: 133–58

Cameron F (1994) Models of specialist practice. In: Humphris D ed. *The Clinical Nurse Specialist: Issues in Practice*. Macmillan, London: 16–28

Castledine G (2003) The development of advanced nursing practice in the UK. In: McGee P, Castledine G, eds. *Advanced Nursing Practice*, 2nd edn. Blackwell, Oxford: 8–16

Castledine G (1998a). Clinical specialists in nursing in the UK: the early years. In: Castledine G, McGee P, eds. *Advanced and Specialist Nursing Practice*. Blackwell Science, Oxford: 3–32

Castledine G (1998b) Clinical specialists in nursing in the UK: 1980s to the present day. In: Castledine G, McGee P, eds. *Advanced and Specialist Nursing Practice*. Blackwell Science, Oxford: 33–54

Castledine G (1996) Encouraging team collaboration in healthcare. *Br J Nurs* **5**(22): 1402

Castledine G (1995a) Defining specialist nursing. *Br J Nurs* **4**(5): 264–65

Castledine G (1995b) Will the nurse practitioner be a mini doctor or a maxi nurse? *Br J Nurs* **4**(16): 938–39

Castledine G (1994). Specialist and advanced nursing and the scope of practice. In: Hunt G, Wainwright P, eds. *Expanding the Role of the Nurse: The Scope of Professional Practice*. Blackwell Scientific, Oxford: 101–13

Castledine G (1991) The advanced nurse practitioner: Part 2. *Nurs Stand* **5**(44): 33–35

Castledine G (1989) The role of the specialist nurse. *RCN Diabetes Nursing Forum Conference Presentation*. Royal College of Nursing, London

Castledine G (1982) The role and function of clinical nurse specialist in England and Wales. Unpublished MSc Thesis, University of Manchester

Castledine G, McGee P, Brown R (1996) *A Survey of Specialist and Advanced Nursing Practice in England*. Nursing Research Unit, University of Central England, Birmingham

Cattell RB (1966) The meaning and strategic use of factor analysis. In: Cattell RB, ed. *Handbook of Multivariate Experimental Psychology*. Rand McNally, Chicago: 174–243

Cattell RB (1992) Handbook of multivariate experimental psychology. Cited in: Stevens J (1992) *Applied Multivariate Statistics for the Social Sciences*, 2nd edn. Lawrence Erlbaum Publishers, Hillsdale: 378–79

Chambers JK, Dangel RB, German K, Tripodi V, Jaeger C (1987) Clinical nurse specialist collaboration: development of a generic job description and standards of performance. *Clin Nurse Spec* **1**(3): 124–27

Christman L (1991) Advanced nursing practice: future of clinical nurse specialists. In: Aiken LH, Fagin CM, eds. *Charting Nursing's Future: Agenda for the 1990s*. JB Lippincott, New York: 108–20

Clarke A (1999) Focus group interviews in health-care research. *Prof Nurse* **14**(6): 395–97

Coffey A, Atkinson P (1996) *Making Sense of Qualitative Data: Complementary Research Strategies*. Sage Publication, Thousand Oaks

Collins EG (1992) Increasing practice-based research: doctorally prepared clinical nurse specialists may be the answer. *Clin Nurse Spec* **6**(4): 196–200

Colomy P, Rhoades G (1983) Role performance and person perception: towards an interactionist approach. *Symbol Interact* **6**(2): 207–27

Conway ME (1988a) Theoretical approaches to the study of roles. In: Hardy ME, Conway ME, eds. *Role Theory: Perspectives for Health Professionals*, 2nd edn. Appleton and Lange, Norwalk: 63–72

Conway ME (1988b) Organisations, professional autonomy, and roles. In: Hardy ME, Conway ME, eds. *Role Theory: Perspectives for Health Professionals*, 2nd edn. Appleton and Lange, Norwalk: 111–32

Cooper DM, Sparacino PSA (1990) Acquiring, implementing, and evaluating the clinical nurse specialist role. In: Sparacino PSA, Cooper DM, Minarik PA, eds. *The Clinical Nurse Specialist: Implementation and Impact*. Appleton and Lange, Norwalk: 41–76

Cradock S (1999) Diabetes: research and nursing. *Pract Diabetes Int* **16**(2): 32

Cradock S (1998) Leadership in diabetes nursing: now is the time to spread our wings. *J Diabetes Nurs* **2**(5): 133–34

Cradock S (1993) Changing role of the clinical nurse specialist. *Diabetes Care* **2**: 5–6

Cradock S (1991) ENB 928. The effect of a diabetes nursing course on diabetes care in the health district. *Diabetic Nurs* **1**: 3–6

Crowley M (2000) Education for diabetes nurses: the challenge for the new millennium. *J Diabetes Nurs* **4**(2): 61–63

Da Costa S (2000) Diabetes specialist nursing: looking to the future, learning from the past. *Br J Nurs* **9**(5): 287–90

Davies B, Hughes AM (1995) Clarification of advanced nursing practice: characteristics and competencies. *Clin Nurse Spec* **9**(3): 156–60; 166

Davis EA (1994) Factors influencing the implementation of the CNS role in a private practice. *Clin Nurse Spec* **8**(1): 42–47

De Witt K (1900) Specialist in nursing. *Am J Nurs* **1**(14): 17

Department of Health (2004) *The NHS Knowledge and Skills Framework (NHS KSF) and Related Development Review*. Department of Health, London

Department of Health (2003). Supplementary prescribing by nurses and pharmacists within the NHS in England: A guide for implementation: *http://www.dh.gov.uk/PublicationsAndStatistics/Publications/PublicationsPolicyAndGuidance/PublicationsPolicyAndGuidanceArticle/fs/en?CONTENT_ID=4009717&chk=11s8x4* (accessed 10.11.2004)

Department of Health (1997) *The New NHS: Modern, Dependable*. HMSO, London

DeVellis RF (1991) *Scale Development: Theory and Applications*. Sage Publications, Newbury Park

Diabetes UK (2000) *Diabetes Specialist Nurse: Directory 2000*. Diabetes UK, London

Dickoff J, James P (1968) A theory of theories: a position paper. *Nurs Res* **17**(3): 197–203

Dickoff J, James P, Wiedenbach E (1997) Theory in a practice discipline. Part II: practice oriented research. In: Nicoll LH, ed. *Perspectives on Nursing Theory*, 3rd edn. Lippincott, Philadelphia: 665–78

Edlund BJ, Hodges LC (1983) Preparing and using the clinical nurse specialist. *Nurs Clin N Am* **18**(3): 499–507

Elkin F, Handel G (1989) *The Child and Society: The Process of Socialisation*, 5th edn. Random House, New York

Farmer G (2000) Evaluation of DSN support to practice nurses. *J Diabetes Nurs* **4**(4): 121–26

Fawcett J (1997). The relationship between theory and research: a double helix. In: Nicoll LH, eds. *Perspectives on Nursing Theory*, 3rd edn. Lippincott, Philadelphia: 716–26

Fawcett J, Downs FS (1992) *The Relationship of Theory and Research*, 2nd edn. FA Davis, Philadelphia

Felton AM (1989) The role of the nurse specialist in diabetes. *Diabetes Nurs* **1**(1): 9–10

Fenton MV (1985) Identifying competencies of clinical nurse specialists. *J Nurs Admin* **15**(12): 31–37

Field A (2000) *Discovering Statistics Using SPSS for Windows: Advanced Techniques for the Beginner*. Sage Publications, London

Frese M (1984) Transitions in jobs, occupational socialisation and strain. In: Allen VL, van de Vliert E, eds. *Role Transitions: Explorations and Explanations*. Plenum Press, New York: 239–52

Froggatt K, Hoult L, Poole K (2001) *Community Work with Nursing and Residential Care Homes: A Survey Study of Clinical Nurse Specialists in Palliative Care*. Macmillan Cancer Research, London

Gaines KA (1981) Role expectations for the hospital-employed clinical nurse specialist. Unpublished DSN Thesis, University of Alabama in Birmingham, USA

Georgopoulos B, Christman L (1970) The clinical nurse specialist: a role model. *Am J Nurs* **70**(5): 1030–39

Gerrish CA (1990) An analysis of the educational role of the ward sister (implications for nurse educators). *Nurse Educ Today* **10**: 198–205

Gibson F, Bamford O (2001) Focus group interviews to examine the role and development of the clinical nurse specialist. *J Nurs Manage* **9**: 331–42

Girard N (1987) The CNS: development of the role. In: Menard SW, eds. *The Clinical Nurse Specialist: Perspectives on Practice*. John Wiley and Sons, New York: 9–36

Girouard S (1983) Theory-based practice: functions, obstacles, and solutions. In: Hamric AB, Spross J, eds. *The Clinical Nurse Specialist in Theory and Practice*. Grune and Stratton, Orlando: 39–57

Goode WJ (1966) Norm commitment and conformity to role-status obligations. In: Biddle BJ, Thomas EJ, eds. *Role Theory: Concepts and Research*. John Wiley and Sons, New York: 313–18

Goodwin M, Higgins S, Lenfear JH, Lewis S, Winterbottom J (2004) The role of the clinical nurse specialist in epilepsy. A notional survey. *Seizure* **13**: 87–94

Graen G (1976) Role-making processes within complex organisations. In: Dunnette M, ed. *Handbook of Industrial and Organisational Psychology*. Rand-McNally, Chicago

Griffiths J, Luker K (1994) Community nurse attitudes to the clinical nurse specialist. *Nurs Times* **90**(17): 39–42

Gross N, Mason WS, McEachern AW (1958) *Explorations in Role Analysis: Studies in the School Superintendency Role*. Wiley, New York

Halsey S (1978) The Queen Bee Syndrome: one solution to role conflict for nurse managers. In: Hardy ME, Conway ME, eds. *Role Theory: Perspectives for Health Professionals*. Appleton-Century-Crofts, New York: 231–50

Halvatsiotis P, Raptis AE, Anastasiou E, Tsapogas P, Boutati E, Raptis SA (2000) *The Hellenic National Diabetes Network and the Diabetes Healthcare Medical Record*. Paper presented in the 7th DOIT Workshop, Gubbio-Italy, 12–14 May 2000

Hamric AB (2005) A definition of advanced practice nursing. In: Hamric AB, Spross JA, Hanson CM, eds. *Advanced Practice Nursing: An Integrative Approach*, 3rd edn. Elsevier Saunders, Philadelphia, PA: 85–108

Hamric AB (1998) Historical and current development in specialist and advanced practice in North America. In: Castledine G, McGee P, eds. *Advanced and Specialist Nursing Practice*. Blackwell Science, Oxford: 55–70

Hamric AB (1992). Creating our future: challenges and opportunities for the clinical nurse specialist. *Oncol Nurs Forum* **19**(1): 11–15

Hamric AB (1989) History and overview of the CNS role. In: Hamric AB, Spross JA, eds. *The Clinical Nurse Specialist in Theory and Practice*, 2nd edn. WB Saunders, Philadelphia: 3–18

Hamric AB (1983) Role development and functions. In: Hamric AB, Spross JA, eds. *The Clinical Nurse Specialist in Theory and Practice*. Grune and Stratton, Orlando: 39–56

Hamric AB, Hanson CM (2003) Educating advanced practice nurses for practice reality. *J Prof Nurs* **19**(5): 262–68

Hamric AB, Reigle J (2005) Ethical decision making. In: Hamric AB, Spross JA, Hanson CM, eds. *Advanced Practice Nursing: An Integrative Approach*, 3rd edn. Elsevier Saunders, St Louis

Hamric AB, Spross JA (1989) *The Clinical Nurse Specialist in Theory and Practice*, 2nd edn. WB Saunders, Philadelphia

Hamric AB, Taylor J (1989) Role development of the CNS. In: Hamric AB, Spross JA, eds. *The Clinical Nurse Specialist in Theory and Practice*, 2nd edn. WB Saunders, Philadelphia: 41–82

Hanson CM, Malone BL (2000) Leadership: empowerment, change agency and activism. In: Hamric AB, Spross JA, Hanson CM, eds. *Advanced Nursing Practice: An Integrative Approach*, 2nd edn. WB Saunders, Philadelphia: 279–313

Hanson CM, Spross JA, Carr DB (2000) Collaboration. In: Hamric AB, Spross JA, Hanson CM, eds. *Advanced Nursing Practice: An Integrative Approach*, 2nd edn. WB Saunders, Philadelphia: 315–47

Hardy ME (1978a) Perspectives on knowledge and role theory. In: Hardy ME, Conway ME, eds. *Role Theory: Perspectives for Health Professionals*. Appleton-Century-Crofts, New York: 1–15

Hardy ME (1978b) Role stress and role strain. In: Hardy ME, Conway ME, eds. *Role Theory: Perspectives for Health Professionals*. Appleton-Century-Crofts, New York: 73 – 109

Hardy ME (1988) Perspectives on science. In: Hardy ME, Conway ME, eds. *Role Theory: Perspectives for Health Professionals,* 2nd edn. Appleton and Lange, Norwalk: 1–27

Hardy ME, Conway ME (1988) *Role Theory: Perspectives for Health Professionals*, 2nd edn. Appleton and Lange, Norwalk

Hardy ME, Hardy WL (1988a) Development of scientific knowledge. In: Hardy ME, Conway ME, eds. *Role Theory: Perspectives for Health Professionals,* 2nd edn. Appleton and Lange, Norwalk: 29–62

Hardy ME, Hardy WL (1988b) Role stress and role strain. In: Hardy ME, Conway ME, eds. *Role Theory: Perspectives for Health Professionals,* 2nd edn. Appleton and Lange, Norwalk: 241–56

Hardy ME, Conway ME (1978) *Role Theory: Perspectives for Health Professionals.* Appleton-Century-Crofts, New York

Harrell JS, McCulloch SD (1986) The role of the clinical nurse specialist: problems and solutions. *J Nurs Admin* **16**(10): 44–48

Haste F, MacDonald LD (1992) The role of the specialist in community nursing: perceptions of specialist and district nurses. *Int J Nurs Stud* **29**(1): 37–47

Hellenic DoH (1990) *Requirements on Structure and Organisation of Diabetes Outpatients Clinics and Diabetes Centres of Public Hospitals.* Department of Health, Athens [Greek]

Hellman C (1974). The making of a clinical specialist. *Nurs Outlook* **22**(3): 165–67

Holle ML, Blatchley ME (1989) Teaching leadership with role theory. *Nurs Conn* **2**(4): 53–61

Holt FM (1987) Executive practice: developmental stages of the clinical nurse specialist role. *Clin Nurse Spec* **1**(3): 116–18

Holt FM (1984) A theoretical model for clinical specialist practice. *Nurs Health Care* **5**(8): 445–49

Humphris D (1994a) *The Clinical Nurse Specialist: Issues in Practice.* Macmillan, London

Humphris D (1994b) The basis of role specialism in nursing. In: Humphris D, ed. *Clinical Nurse Specialist: Issues in Practice.* Macmillan, London: 1–15

Humphris D, Hamilton S, O'Halloran P, Fisher S, Littlejohns P (1999) Do diabetes nurse specialists utilise research evidence? *Practical Diabetes Int* **16**(2): 47–50

Hurley-Wilson BA (1988) Socialisation for roles. In: Hardy ME, Conway ME, eds. *Role theory: Perspectives for Health Professionals*, 2nd edn. Appleton and Lange, Norwalk: 73–110

International Council of Nurses (1992) *Guidelines on Specialisation in Nursing.* International Council of Nurses, Geneva

International Diabetes Federation (2000) *Diabetes Atlas 2000.* International Diabetes Federation, Brussels

Jackson J (1998a) Contemporary criticisms of role theory. *J Occup Sci* **5**(2): 49–55

Jackson P (1998b) Focus group interviews as a methodology. *Nurse Researcher* **6**(1): 72–84

James J (2004) Supplementary prescribing by a diabetes specialist nurse on a hospital ward. *Nurse Prescribing* **2**(3): 112–16

Johns P (1997) Activity analysis on the workload of the diabetes specialist nurse. *J Diabetes Nurs* **1**(2): 50–53

Johnson DE (1962) Consequences for patients and personnel. *Am J Nurs* **62**: 96–100

Kahn RL, Wolfe DM, Quinn RP, Snoek JD, Rosenthal RA (1981) *Organisational Stress: Studies in Role Conflict and Ambiguity*, reprint. Robert E Krieger Publishing, Malabar, FL

Kaiser H F (1960) The application of electronic computers to factor analysis. *Educ Psycholog Measur* **20**: 141–51. Cited in: Stevens J (1992) *Applied Multivariate Statistics for the Social Sciences*, 2nd edn. Lawrence Erlbaum Associates, Hillsdale: 378

Katz D, Kahn R (1978) *The Social Psychology of Organisation*, 2nd edn. John Wiley and Sons, New York

Keeling AW, Bigbee JL (2005). The history of advanced practice nursing in the United States. In: Hamric AB, Spross JA, Hanson CM, eds. *Advanced Practice Nursing: An Integrative Approach*, 3rd edn. Elsevier Saunders, St Louis: 3–45

Kelly J (1982) Role theory as a model for human interaction: its implications for nursing education. *Aus Nurse J* **12**(1): 42–43; 51

Kerrison S (1990) *A Diplomat in the Job: Diabetes Nursing and the Changing Division of Labour in Diabetic Care.* Research Paper 4. Health and Social Services Unit, Southbank Polytechnic, London: 12–19

King MB (1990) Clinical nurse specialist collaboration with physicians. *Clin Nurse Spec* **4**(4): 172–77

Kinson J, Nattrass M (1984) *Caring for the Diabetic Patient.* Churchill Livingstone, Edinburgh

Kitzinger J, Barbour RS (1999) Introduction: the challenge and promise of focus groups. In: Barbour RS, Kitzinger J, eds. *Developing Focus Group Research: Politics, Theory and Practice.* Sage Publications, London: 1–20

Klein DG (1994) Critical care clinical nurse specialist: novice to expert. In: Gawlinski A, Kern LS, eds. *The Clinical Nurse Specialist Role in critical care.* WB Saunders, Philadelphia: 24–39

Kline P (2000) *Handbook of Psychological Testing*, 2nd edn. Routledge, London

Kline P (1994) *An Easy Guide to Factor Analysis.* Routledge, London

Koetters TL (1989) Clinical practice and direct patient care. In: Hamric AB, Spross JA, eds. *The Clinical Nurse Specialist in Theory and Practice*, 2nd edn. W B Saunders, Philadelphia: 107–23

Kramer M (1974) *Reality Shock: Why Nurses Leave Nursing*. Mosby, St Louis

Kumar R (1996) *Research Methodology: A Step-by-Step Guide for Beginners*. Sage Publications, London

Kyne-Grzebalski D (1997) The role of the diabetes specialist nurse. In: Pickup J, Williams G, eds. *Textbook of Diabetes*, 2nd edn. Blackwell Scientific, Oxford: 81.1–81.8

Lancaster J (1982) Change theory: an essential aspect of nursing practice. In: Lancaster J, Lancaster W, eds. *The Nurse as a Change Agent*. CV Mosby, St Louis: 3–28

Leddy S, Pepper JM (1989) *Conceptual Bases of Professional Practice*, 2nd edn. JB Lippincott, Philadelphia

Lemonidou C (1999) The role of the nurse in the care of people with diabetes. *Nosileftiki* **2**: 174–80 [Greek]

Lillyman S (1998) Assessing competence. In: Castledine G, McGee P, eds. *Advanced and Specialist Nursing Practice*. Blackwell Science, Oxford: 119–31

Linton R (1936) *The Study of Man: An Introduction*. Appleton-Century, New York

Llahana SV, Gerogianni GK (2003) Exploring the role of the diabetes specialist nurse: role components and activities. *Nosileftiki* **42**(1): 82–96 [Greek]

Llahana SV, Poulton BC, Coates VE (2001a) The paediatric diabetes specialist nurse and diabetes education in childhood. *J Adv Nurs* **33**(3): 296–306

Llahana SV, Poulton BC, Coates VE (2001b) Role development of the diabetes specialist nurse: a pilot study. *J Diabetes Nurs* **5**(4): 114–18

Loewenthal KM (2001) *An Introduction to Psychological Tests and Scales*, 2nd edn. Psychology Press, East Sussex

Loudermilk L (1990). Role ambiguity and the clinical nurse specialist. *Nurs Conn* **3**(1): 3–12

MacKinnon M (1998a) *Providing Diabetes Care in General Practice: A Practical Guide for the Primary Care Team*, 3rd edn. Class Publishing, London

MacKinnon M (1998b) The future role of the diabetes specialist nurse. *J Diabetes Nurs* **2**(3): 68–69

Major DA (2003) Utilizing role theory to help employed parents cope with children's chronic illness. *Health Educ Res* **18**(1): 45–57

Malone B (1986) Evaluation of the clinical nurse specialist. *Am J Nurs* **86**(12): 1375–77

Marshall Z, Luffingham N (1998) Does the specialist nurse enhance or deskill the general nurse? *Br J Nurs* **7**(11): 658–62

Masterson A, Mitchell L (2003) Developing competence for advanced practice. In: McGee P, Castledine G, eds. *Advanced Nursing Practice*, 2nd edn. Blackwells, Oxford: 31–46

McCaffrey-Boyle D (1997) Lessons learned from clinical nurse specialist longevity. *J Adv Nurs* **26**: 1168–74

McCaffrey-Boyle D (1996) The clinical nurse specialist. In: Hamric AB, Spross JA, Hanson CM, eds. *Advanced Nursing Practice: An Integrative Approach*. WB Saunders, Philadelphia: 299–336

McDaniel RW, Bach CA (1996) Focus group research: The question of scientific rigor. *Rehab Nurs Res* **5**(2): 53–59

McFadden EA, Miller MA (1994) Clinical nurse specialist practice: facilitators and barriers. *Clin Nurse Spec* **8**(1): 27–33

McGarvey HE (1998) The Operating Department: Investigating the Role of the Nurse. Unpublished Thesis (PhD), University of Ulster, N Ireland

McGee P (1998) Specialist practice in the UK. In: Castledine G, McGee P, eds. *Advanced and Specialist Nursing Practice*. Blackwell Science, Oxford: 135–45

McGee P, Castledine G (1999) A survey of specialist and advanced nursing practice in the UK. *Br J Nurs* **8**(16): 1074–78

McGee P, Castledine G (1998). *A Survey of Specialist and Advanced Nursing Practice in the United Kingdom*. Nursing Research Unit, University of Central England, Birmingham:

McGuire DB, Harwood KV (2000). Research. In: Hamric AB, Spross JA, Hanson CM, eds. *Advanced Nursing Practice: An Integrative Approach*, 2nd edn. WB Saunders, Philadelphia: 217–43

McKenna H (1997) *Nursing Theories and Models: Essentials for Nurses*. Routledge, London

McLafferty I (2004) Focus group interviews as a data collecting strategy. *J Adv Nurs* **48**(2): 187–94

Mead GH (1934) *Mind, Self and Society: From the Standpoint of a Social Behaviourist*. University of Chicago Press, Chicago

Meleis AI (1975) Role sufficiency and role supplementation: a conceptual framework. *Nurs Res* **24**(4): 264–71

Menard SW (1987a) *The Clinical Nurse Specialist: Perspectives on Practice*. John Wiley and Sons, New York

Menard SW (1987b) The CNS as practitioner. In: Menard SW, eds. *The Clinical Nurse Specialist: Perspectives on Practice*. John Wiley and Sons, New York: 81–100

Merton RK (1968) *Social Theory and Social Structure*. Free Press, New York

Miller S (1995) The clinical nurse specialist: a way forward. *J Adv Nurs* **22**: 494–501

Moody LE (1990) *Advancing Nursing Science Through Research*, Vol 1. Sage Publications, Newbury Park

Moore WE (1969) Occupational socialisation. In: Goslin DA, eds. *Handbook of Socialisation Theory and Research*. Rand McNally College Publishing, Chicago: 861–83

Morath J (1988) The CSN: evaluation issues. *Nurs Manage* **19**(3): 72–80

Moreno JL (1960) *The Sociometry Reader*. Free Press, Glencoe, Ill

Moreno JL (1934) *Who Shall Survive? A New Approach to the Problem of Human Interrelations*. Nervous and Mental Disease Publishing, Washington, DC

Muldoon-Mastey J, Cole FL (1992) A theoretic perspective on postcode stress experienced by critical care nurses. *Heart Lung* **21**(3): 208–13

Nash A (1991) Working with specialists. *J District Nurs* **10**(6): 8–11

National Association of Clinical Nurse Specialists (2004) *Statement on Clinical Nurse Specialist Practice and Education*. Author, Harrisburg, PA

Naylor MD, Brooten D (1993) The roles and functions of clinical nurse specialists. *Image: J Nurs Schol* **25**: 73–78

Newton J, Waters V (2001) Community palliative care clinical nurse specialists' descriptions of stress in their work. *Int J Pall Nurs* **7**(11): 531–40

Nightingale F (1859) *Notes on Nursing: What It Is and What It Is Not* (reprinted 1970). Churchill Livingstone, Edinburgh

Noone J (1987) Planned change: putting theory into practice. *Clin Nurse Spec* **1**(1): 25–29

Nuccio SA, Costa-Lieberthal KM, Gunta KE, *et al* (1993) A survey of 636 staff nurses: perceptions and factors influencing the CNS role. *Clin Nurse Spec* **7**(3): 122–28

Nunnally JC, Bernstein IH (1994) *Psychometric Theory*, 3rd edn. McGraw-Hill, New York

O'Keeffe B, Gillis CL (1988) Family care in the coronary care unit: An analysis of clinical nurse specialist intervention. *Heart Lung* **17**: 191–98

O'Rourke MW (1989) Generic professional behaviours: implications for the clinical nurse specialist role. *Clin Nurse Spec* **3**(3): 128–32

Oda D (1977) Specialised role development: a three-phase process. *Nurs Outlook* **25**(6): 374–77

Oda D, Sparacino PS, Boyd P (1988) Role advancement for the experienced clinical nurse specialist. *Clin Nurse Spec* **2**(4): 167–71

Oddi LF, Cassidy VR (1998) The message of SUPPORT: Change is long overdue. *J Prof Nurs* **14**(3): 165–74

Oeser OA, Harary F (1966) Role structures: a description in terms of graph theory. In: Biddle BJ, Thomas EJ, eds. *Role Theory: Concepts and Research*. John Wiley & Sons, New York: 92–102

Oppenheim AN (1992) *Questionnaire Design, Interviewing and Attitude Measurement*. Pinter Publishers, London

Padmore E (2000) Higher level nursing: influencing care at all levels of the organisation. *J Diabetes Nurs* **4**(3): 74–77

Page NE, Arena DM (1991) Practical strategies for clinical nurse specialist role implementation. *Clin Nurse Spec* **5**(1): 43–48

Parahoo K (1997) *Nursing Research: Principles, Process and Issues*. Macmillan, London

Parker S (1997) The implications of autonomy for the diabetes specialist nurse. *J Diabetes Nurs* **1**(1): 22–24

Parsons T (1966) Role conflict and the genesis of deviance. In: Biddle BJ, Thomas EJ, eds. *Role theory: Concepts and Research*. John Wiley & Sons, New York: 275–76

Patterson C, Haddad B (1992) The advanced nurse practitioner: common attributes. *Can J Nurs Admin* **5**(3): 18–22

Polit DF, Beck CT, Hungler BP (2001) *Essentials of Nursing Research: Methods, Appraisal and Utilisation*, 5th edn. Lippincott, Philadelphia

Polit DF, Hungler BP (1999) *Nursing Research: Principles and Methods*, 6th edn. Lippincott, Philadelphia

Powell J (1989) The reflective practitioner in nursing. *J Adv Nurs* **14**: 824–32

Powell RA, Single HM (1996) Focus groups. *Int J Qual Health Care* **8**(5): 499–504

Priest AR (1989) The CNS as educator. In: Hamric AB, Spross JA, eds. *The Clinical Nurse Specialist in Theory and Practice*, 2nd edn. WB Saunders, Philadelphia: 147–67

Ray GL, Hardin S (1995) Advanced practice nursing: playing a vital role. *Nurs Manage* 26: 45–47

Redmond S (1988) *Diabetes Specialist Nurses and Training Questionnaire*. Diabetes UK, London

Reigle J, Boyle RJ (2000) Ethical decision-making skills. In: Hamric AB, Spross JA, Hanson CM, eds. *Advanced Nursing Practice: An Integrative Approach*, 2nd edn. WB Saunders, Philadelphia: 349–79

Reiskin H (1992) Focus groups: A useful technique for research and practice in nursing. *Appl Nurs Res* **5**(4): 197–201

Reiter F (1966) The nurse clinician. *Am J Nurs* **66**: 274–80

Richmond J (2004) General nurses' perceptions of the role of the clinical nurse specialist in Ireland. *Cancer Nurs Pract* **3**(6): 33–39

Riggin OZ (1982) Role theory and nursing practice. In: Lancaster J, Lancaster W, eds. *The Nurse as a Change Agent*. CV Mosby, St Louis: 65–78

Robichaud AM, Hamric AB (1986). Time documentation of clinical nurse specialist activities. *J Nurs Admin* **16**(1): 31–36

Robinson N (1999) The use of focus group methodology—with selected examples from sexual health research. *J Adv Nurs* **29**(4): 905–13

Rodgers-Ward C (1986) The meaning of role strain. *Adv Nurs Sci* **8**(2): 39–49

Rosse JG, Rosse PH (1981) Role conflict and ambiguity: An empirical investigation of nursing personnel. *Eval Health Professions* **4**: 385–405

Royal College of Nursing (1991) *Diabetes Nursing Forum Working Party Report: The Role of the Diabetes Specialist Nurse*. Royal College of Nursing, London

Royal College of Nursing (1988) *Specialties in Nursing: A Report of the Working Party Investigating the Development of Specialties within the Nursing Profession*. Royal College of Nursing, London

Rubin S (1988) The expanded role nurse, part II. Role implementation strategies. *Can J Nurs Admin* **1**(3): 12–15

Ryan-Merritt MV, Mitchell R, Pagel I (1988) Clinical nurse specialist: role definition and operationalisation. *Clin Nurse Spec* **2**(3): 132–37

Sarbin T, Allen VL (1968) Role theory. In: Lindsey G, Aronson E, Eds. *The Handbook of Social Psychology*, 2nd edn. Addison-Wesley, Reading: 488–568

Scherer YK, Jezewski MA, Janelli LM, Ackerman MA, Ludwig MA (1994) Nursing administrators' perceptions of critical care clinical nurse specialists. *Clin Nurse Spec* **8**: 138–44; 151

Scott RA (1999) A description of the roles, activities, and skills of clinical specialists in the United States. *Clin Nurse Spec* **13**(4): 183–90

Scott RA (1997) Identifying the roles, activities, skills, and the cost-saving and revenue-generating activities of Masters prepared nurses who function in traditional clinical nurse specialist roles in the United States. Unpublished PhD Thesis, Georgia State University, Atlanta

Scott W (1970) *Social Processes and Social Structures: An Introduction to Sociology*. Holt, Rinehart and Winston, New York

Simpson IH (1979) *From Student to Nurse: A Longitudinal Study of Socialisation*. Cambridge University Press, Cambridge

Snyder M (1989) Educational preparation of the CNS. In: Hamric A B, Spross JA, eds. The Clinical Nurse Specialist in Theory and Practice, 2nd edn. WB Saunders, Philadelphia: 325–42

Sokol M, Louis MR (1984) Career transitions and life event adaptation: integrating alternative perspectives on role transition. In: Allen VL, van de Vliert E, eds. *Role Transitions: Explorations and Explanations*. Plenum Press, New York: 81–94

Sparacino PSA (2005) The clinical nurse specialist. In: Hamric AB, Spross JA, Hanson CM. eds. *Advanced Practice Nursing: An Integrative Approach*, 3rd edn. Elsevier Saunders, St Louis: 415–46

Sparacino PSA (2000) The Clinical Nurse Specialist. In: Hamric AB, Spross JA, Hanson CM, eds. *Advanced Nursing Practice: An Integrative Approach*, 2nd edn. WB Saunders, Philadelphia: 381–405

Sparacino PSA (1990) A historical perspective on the development of the clinical nurse specialist role. In: Sparacino PSA, Cooper DM, Minarik PA, eds. *The Clinical Nurse Specialist: Implementation and Impact*. Appleton and Lange, Norwalk: 3–10

Sparacino PSA (1986) The clinical nurse specialist. In: Holzemer WL, eds. *Review of Research in Nursing Education*, Vol 1. National League for Nursing, New York: 165–88

Sparacino PSA, Cooper DM (1990) The role components. In: Sparacino PSA, Cooper DM, Minarik PA, eds. *The Clinical Nurse Specialist: Implementation and Impact*. Appleton and Lange, Norwalk: 11–40

Spross JA (1989) The CNS as collaborator. In: Hamric AB, Spross JA, eds. *The Clinical Nurse Specialist in Theory and Practice*, 2nd edn. WB Saunders, Philadelphia: 205–25

Spross JA, Clarke EB, Beauregard J (2000) Expert coaching and guidance. In: Hamric A B, Spross JA, Hanson C M, eds. *Advanced Nursing Practice: An Integrative Approach*, 2nd edn. WB Saunders, Philadelphia: 299–336

Sterling YM, McNally JA (1999) Clinical practice of doctorally prepared nurses. *Clin Nurse Spec* **13**(6): 296–302

Stetler C, DiMaggio G (1991) Research utilisation among clinical nurse specialists. *Clin Nurse Spec* **5**: 151–55

Stevens BJ (1976) Accountability of the clinical specialist: an administrator's viewpoint. *J Nurs Admin* **6**(2): 30–32

Stevens J (1992) *Applied Multivariate Statistics for the Social Sciences*, 2nd edn. Lawrence Erlbaum Associates, Hillsdale

Stewart DW, Shamdasani PN (1990) *Focus Groups: Theory and Practice*. Sage Publications, Newbury Park

Storr G (1988) The clinical nurse specialist: from the outside looking in. *J Adv Nurs* **13**(2): 265–72

Tabachnick BG, Fidell LS (1989) *Using Multivariate Statistics*, 2nd edn. Harper Collins, New York:

Tarsitano B, Brophy E, Snyder D (1986) A demystification of the clinical nurse specialist's role. Perceptions of clinical nurse specialists and nurse administrators. *J Nurs Educ* **25**(1): 4–9

Thomas EJ, Biddle BJ (1966a) The nature and history of role theory. In: Biddle BJ, Thomas EJ, eds. *Role Theory: Concepts and Research.* John Wiley and Sons, New York: 3–19

Thomas EJ, Biddle BJ (1966b) Basic concepts for the variables of role phenomena. In: Biddle, BJ, Thomas EJ, eds. *Role Theory: Concepts and Research.* John Wiley and Sons, New York: 51–63

Topham DL (1987) Role theory in relation to roles of the clinical nurse specialist. *Clin Nurse Spec* **1**(2): 81–84

Turner C (1987) Educated for practice: the diabetes nurse specialist. *Senior Nurse* **7**(5): 28–29

Turner JH (1991) *The Structure of Sociological Theory*, 5th edn. Wadsworth Publishing, Belmont, CA

Turner RH (1966) Role-taking, role standpoint, and reference-group behaviour. In: Biddle BJ, Thomas EJ, eds. *Role Theory: Concepts and Research.* John Wiley and Sons, New York: 151–59

Twinn S (1998) An analysis of the effectiveness of focus groups as a method of qualitative data collection with Chinese populations in nursing research. *J Adv Nurs* **28**(3): 654–61

United Kingdom Central Council (1998) *Standards for Specialist Education and Practice. Nursing and Midwifery Council*, London

United Kingdom Central Council (1994) *The Future of Professional Practice—The Council's Standards for Education and Practice following Registration. Position Statement on Policy and Implementation, March 1994.* United Kingdom Central Council, London

United Kingdom Central Council (1992a) *The Scope of Professional Practice: A UKCC Position Statement.* Nursing and Midwifery Council, London

United Kingdom Central Council (1992b) *Code of Professional Conduct.* Nursing and Midwifery Council, London

United Kingdom Central Council (1990) *The Report of Post-Registration Education and Practice Project.* Nursing and Midwifery Council, London

Utz SW, Gleit CJ (1995) Current developments in research-based interventions: enhancing and advancing the CNS role. *Clin Nurse Spec* **9**(1): 8–11; 22

Vick C, Gardner P (2000) Nurse prescribers: are they already out there? *J Diabetes Nurs* **4**(6): 179–82

Wade B, Moyer A (1989) An evaluation of clinical nurse specialists: implications for education and the organisation of care. *Senior Nurse* **9**(9): 11–16

Walker JB (1953) Fieldwork of a diabetic clinic. *Lancet* **2**: 445–47

Walker M (1986) How nursing service administrators view clinical nurse specialists? *Nurs Man* **17**(3): 52–54

Wallace M, Correy L (1983) The clinical specialist as manager: myth versus realities. *J Nurs Admin* **13**(6): 13–15

Wallymahmed M (1997) Practical advice for new diabetes specialist nurses. *Practical Diabetes* **7**(6): 269–72

Watkinson M (2000a) Clinical experience matters. *J Diabetes Nurs* **4**(1): 4

Watkinson M (2000b) Do we really need diabetes degrees? *J Diabetes Nurs* **4**(3): 68–69

Watkinson M (1998) Diabetes specialist nursing: a vision for the future. *J Diabetes Nurs* **2**(3): 86–89

Watkinson M (1997) How do you define a diabetes specialist nurse? *J Diabetes Nurs* **1**(3): 68–69

White R (1977) Mature or matutinal. *Nurs Mirror* **144**(16): 41

Williams A (1993) Steps to develop a working relationship: an evaluation of the community-based clinical nurse specialist. *Professional Nurse* **8**: 806–12

Winch AE (1989) Peer support and peer review. In: Hamric AB, Spross JA, eds. *The Clinical Nurse Specialist in Theory and Practice*, 2nd edn. WB Saunders, Philadelphia: 299–321

Winocour PH, Ford M, Ainsworth A (2002) Association of British Clinical Diabetologists (ABCD): survey of specialist diabetes services in the UK, 2000. 2. workforce issues, roles and responsibilities of diabetes specialist nurses. *Diabetic Med* **19**(Suppl. 4): 27–31

Workshop Report (1990) Diabetes care and research in Europe: the Saint Vincent Declaration. *Diabetic Med* **7**: 360

Worth-Butler M, Murphy R, Fraser D (1994) Towards an integrated model of competence. *Midwifery* **10**: 225–31

Yallop J (1998) A service with quality: helping more nurses get into research. *J Diabetes Nurs* **2**(4): 119–21

Young ME (1988) Entering the system as a clinical specialist using the medium of the patient care conference. *Clin Nurse Specialist* **2**: 138–42

Index

Printed in the United Kingdom
by Lightning Source UK Ltd.
106242UKS00002B/51-60